# Handbook of

# Retinal Disease

## A Case-Based Approach

# Handbook of

# Retinal Disease

## A Case-Based Approach

**Elias Reichel MD**
Professor of Ophthalmology
Department of Ophthalmology, New England Eye Center
Tufts University School of Medicine
Boston, Massachusetts, USA

**Jay S Duker MD**
Director, New England Eye Center
Professor and Chairman of Ophthalmology, Tufts Medical Center
Tufts University School of Medicine
Boston, Massachusetts, USA

**Darin R Goldman MD**
Vitreoretinal Surgeon, Retina Group of Florida
Boca Raton, Florida, USA

**Robin A Vora MD**
Chief of Ophthalmology
Medical Retina and Cataract Surgery
Department of Ophthalmology, The Permanente Medical Group
Oakland, California, USA

**Jordana G Fein MD MS**
Assistant Professor of Ophthalmology
Department of Ophthalmology, Tufts Medical Center
Boston, Massachusetts, USA

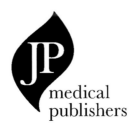

JP
medical
publishers

London • Philadelphia • Panama City • New Delhi

ISBN: 978-1-907816-92-5

**British Library Cataloguing in Publication Data**
A catalogue record for this book is available from the British Library

**Library of Congress Cataloging in Publication Data**
A catalog record for this book is available from the Library of Congress

| | |
|---|---|
| Publisher: | Geoff Greenwood |
| Development Editor: | Gavin Smith |
| Editorial Assistant | Katie Pattullo |
| Design: | Designers Collective Ltd |

Typeset, printed and bound in India.

# Preface

During medical training, caring for patients with complex diseases often involves multi-disciplinary educational gatherings. In the field of ophthalmology, and the retinal sub-specialty specifically, these activities include grand rounds, retinal imaging conferences, and other case-based interactions. After medical training concludes, the majority of practitioners leave the academic setting for general clinical practice and these 'high-yield' multi-disciplinary learning opportunities become far less frequent. However, the variety and complexity of diseases that an ophthalmologist may encounter remains diverse. In daily practice, it becomes more challenging to maintain up to date knowledge regarding both complex and more common retinal diseases, specifically related to characteristic diagnostic findings, current imaging modalities, and treatment.

The aim of this book is to provide a 'high-yield', easily accessible educational reference, while also offering the sense of an interactive case-based conference. We want each chapter to allow the reader to re-construct the sense of a grand rounds or retinal imaging conference. The book is divided into sections based on general retinal disease categories. Within a section, each chapter is devoted to a single diagnosis, ranging from simple to complex. The cases simulate a real patient presenting with a complaint or finding typical of the disease. The reader is then guided through the process of determining the key pathologic clinical finding, formulating a stratified differential diagnosis, asking pertinent historical questions, and determining appropriate diagnostic testing to achieve the correct diagnosis. The condition in question is then discussed in detail with an emphasis on critical diagnostic clinical and imaging findings.

*Handbook of Retinal Disease: A Case-Based Approach* was written with the notion that physicians are perpetual students, always looking for an opportunity to further their knowledge and remain current. However, finding time to stay up to date remains a significant challenge to the average practitioner. The unique format of our book provides an effective yet efficient method to stay current on retinal diseases in a case-based layout. We hope that this book will be useful to retinal specialists, ophthalmologists with a particular interest in retinal diseases, and ophthalmologists preparing for board examinations. Trainees, including medical students, residents, and fellows will also find it useful.

We hope that this book fills a gap and provides a useful resource to your daily practice.

Elias Reichel
Jay S Duker
Darin R Goldman
Robin A Vora
Jordana G Fein
December 2014

# Contents

## Section 4: Vitreoretinal interface abnormalities and diseases of the vitreous

# Contributors

**Caroline R Baumal MD FRCSC**
Associate Professor of Ophthalmology
Department of Vitreoretinal Surgery
New England Eye Center
Tufts University School of Medicine
Boston, MA
USA

**Sundeep K Kasi MD**
Resident in Ophthalmology
Department of Ophthalmology
University of California, San Francisco
San Francisco, CA
USA

**Michelle C Liang MD**
Vitreoretinal Fellow
New England Eye Center
Tufts Medical Center
Boston, MA
USA

**Nora W Muakkassa MD**
Clinical Associate
Department of Ophthalmology
Tufts Medical Center
Boston, MA
USA

**Lauren S Taney MD**
Medical Retina Fellow
New England Eye Center
Tufts Medical Center
Boston, MA
USA

# Section 1

# Normal retina

## Ancillary diagnostic imaging interpretation

### Optical coherence tomography

A normal optical coherence tomography demonstrates the presence of multiple neural retinal layers including the nerve fiber layer, ganglion cell layer, inner plexiform layer, outer plexiform layer, outer nuclear layer, external limiting membrane, photoreceptor layers, and retinal pigment epithelium. The nerve fiber layer represents the axons of the ganglion cell nuclei. The ganglion cell layer contains nuclei of the ganglion cells, the axons of which become the optic nerve fibers. The inner plexiform layer is the region of synapse between the bipolar cell axons and the dendrites of the ganglion and amacrine cells. The inner nuclear layer contains the nuclei of the bipolar cells. The outer plexiform layer is the region of synapse between the rod and cone projections and the bipolar cells. The outer nuclear layer contains the cell bodies of the rods and cones. The external limiting membrane separates the inner segment portion of the photoreceptors from the cell nucleus. The photoreceptor layer contains both rods and cones. However, the foveola has mostly cones and as a result, the outer retina in this area appears lightly bowed (**Figure 1.1**). The retinal pigment epithelium is a single layer of cuboidal epithelial cells, underneath but in contact with the photoreceptors.

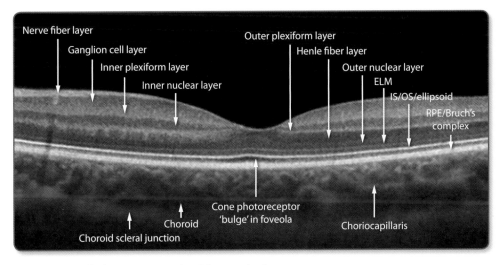

**Figure 1.1** Optical coherence tomography of the normal retina.

## Fluorescein angiography

Fluorescein angiography (FA) examines the circulation of the retina and choroid. FA does not involve the use of ionizing radiation. Fluorescein is injected intravenously and then photographs of the retina are taken using a blue light of 490 nm that causes fluorescence of the dye. There is an exciter filter that allows only blue light of 490 nm to travel to the retina, and a barrier filter, which only allows yellow-green light of 525 nm light to enter the camera (**Figure 1.2**).

In normal patients approximately 10 seconds after the dye is injected, initial choroidal filling (choroidal flush) should be apparent. By 10-12 seconds following injection, the retinal arteries should begin to fill and should completely fill within 1–2 seconds. The early venous stage (laminar venous filling) occurs at 14–15 seconds, with the late venous stage at 18–20 seconds. Normal arteriovenous transit should be no more than 11 seconds. By 5 minutes, late staining may be apparent, which can be used to demonstrate the presence of abnormal vasculature and leakage.

## Indocyanine green angiography

Indocyanine green (ICG) angiography is performed by injecting a cyanine dye intravenously, and allows the visualization of the retinal and choroidal circulation (**Figure 1.3**). ICG has a peak spectral absorption of 800 nm, which is near the infrared range. It penetrates retinal layers allowing for visualization of deeper structures such as the choroidal circulation. ICG can be helpful in evaluation of choroidal masses and diseases such as polypoidal choroidal vasculopathy, central serous chorioretinopathy, and retinal angiomatous proliferation.

## Fundus autofluorescence

Fundus autofluorescence (FAF) is a noninvasive tool to examine the fluorophores of the ocular fundus. A2E within lipofuscin is a naturally occurring fluorophore and appears bright (hyperautofluorescent) (**Figure 1.4**). Other fluorophores include advanced glycation end

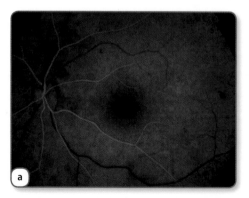
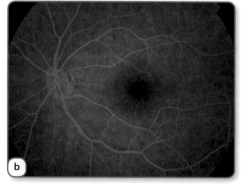

**Figure 1.2** Normal fluorescein angiogram. (a) Early and (b) late frames.

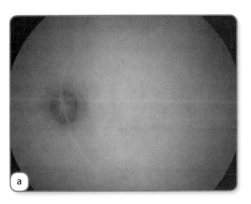 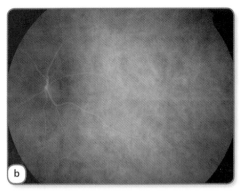

**Figure 1.3** Normal indocyanine green angiography. (a) Early and (b) late frames.

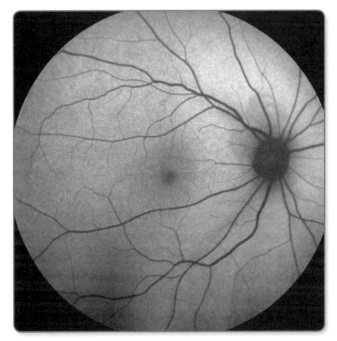

**Figure 1.4** Normal fundus autofluorescence.

products and the redox pair FAD–FADH2, which provides information on retinal energy metabolism. Areas of sick or atrophied retinal pigment epithelium will appear dark (hypoautofluorescent). FAF may be helpful in evaluation of retinal diseases such as age-related macular degeneration, retinitis pigmentosa, central serous retinopathy, pseudoxanthoma elasticum, and macular dystrophies.

## Red-free photography

In red-free photography, the imaging light is filtered to remove red colors, improving contrast of vessels and other structures (**Figure 1.5**).

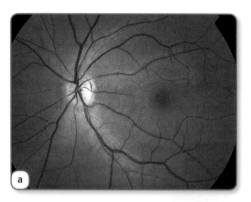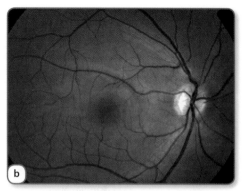

**Figure 1.5** Normal red-free imaging. (a) Right eye. (b) Left eye.

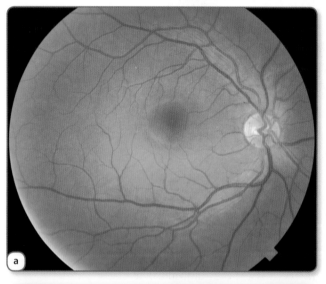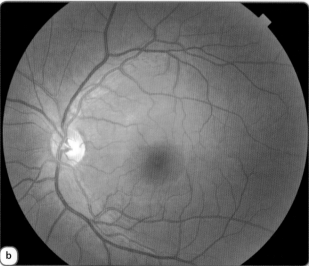

**Figure 1.6** Color fundus photographs. (a) Right eye. (b) Left eye. Note the clear media, normal caliber of vessels and sharp foveal light reflex. There is some mild cup to disc asymmetry between the two eyes, which may be physiologic.

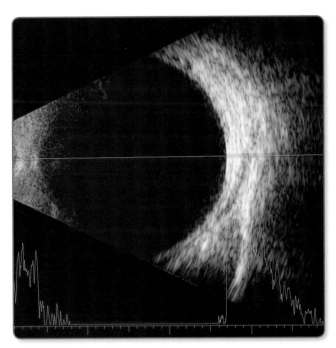

**Figure 1.7** Normal B-scan ultrasound.

It can be helpful for visualization of microaneurysms and hemorrhages, which might be missed clinically.

## Color photography

Normal color photographs should demonstrate the presence of clear media, sharp optic nerve margins without cupping, normal caliber of retinal vessels, and a sharp foveal reflex (**Figure 1.6**).

## B-scan ultrasonography

A B-scan ultrasonography (B scan) uses ultrasound to create a two-dimensional image of the eye (**Figure 1.7**). This is accomplished using high frequency sound waves of 10 mHz that are transmitted from a probe in direct contact with the eye. B scan can be useful when it is not possible to see ocular structures such as the posterior chamber that can occur in the presence of a dense cataract, dense vitreous hemorrhage, or anterior segment opacification. B scan can evaluate for the presence of retinal detachment, choroidal detachment, posterior scleritis, optic nerve head drusen, and choroidal or scleral masses.

# Section 2

# Retinal vascular disease

# Diabetic retinopathy

## How to approach a patient with multiple retinal hemorrhages and cotton-wool spots

| Identify the primary pathologic clinical finding(s) | | |
|---|---|---|
| On examination, the patient may have manifestations of underlying retinal vascular disease like microaneurysms, retinal hemorrhages, retinal lipid exudates, cotton-wool spots, venous beading, capillary nonperfusion, macular edema, and neovascularization. | | |
| **Formulate a differential diagnosis** | | |
| **Most likely** | **Less likely** | **Least likely** |
| • Diabetic retinopathy, radiation retinopathy, hypertensive retinopathy, retinal venous obstruction | • Ocular ischemic syndrome, anemia, leukemia, vasculitis (e.g. lupus and sarcoidosis) | • Coat's disease, idiopathic juxtafoveal telangiectasia, sickle cell retinopathy, medication side effects (interferon) |
| **Query patient history** | | |
| • Does the patient have diabetes, if so for how long? Type I or type II diabetes?<br>• What is the patient's hemoglobin A1c and fasting blood sugar?<br>• What medications is the patient taking?<br>• Is there any other pertinent medical history? (Systemic hypertension, obesity, renal disease, elevated serum lipids, pregnancy)<br>• What is the relevant past ocular history? (Previous injections, lasers, surgery, or trauma) | | |
| **Decide on ancillary diagnostic imaging** | | |
| Diabetic retinopathy is a clinical diagnosis made with ophthalmoscopy. The presence of microaneurysms is the sine qua non. Diabetic macular edema is also a clinical diagnosis; however, optical coherence tomography (OCT) can be used to confirm its presence, as well as identify areas of vitreomacular traction. Fluorescein angiography (FA) with peripheral sweeps can demonstrate macular edema and neovascularization. | | |

## Ancillary diagnostic imaging interpretation

### Color fundus photography

Fundus photography may be useful for documenting substantial progression of disease and response to therapy. It is also used to grade diabetic retinopathy in clinical studies (**Figure 2.1**).

### Optical coherence tomography

OCT can quantify retinal thickness, monitor diabetic macular edema (DME), and identify vitreomacular traction in patients with DME (**Figure 2.2**). OCT is also used to monitor response to therapy. At present, its role as a screening tool for DME is not proven. Macular edema appears as areas of hyporeflectivity due to accumulation of intraretinal and/or subretinal fluid within the outer plexiform layer. OCT may also demonstrate the presence of hard exudates that appear as hyper-reflective spots with shadowing in the outer retinal layers. Identification of 'center-involving' versus 'noncenter involving' DME is a critical step in determining proper therapy.

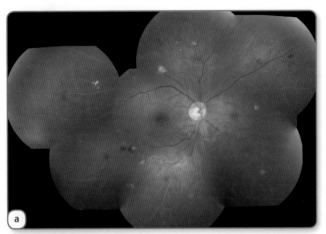

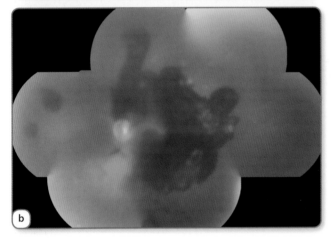

**Figure 2.1** Color mosaic photographs in a patient with proliferative diabetic retinopathy in the right (a) and left eye (b). In (a) note the presence of peripheral nonperfusion with sclerotic vessels. There are also areas of retinal hemorrhages and lipid exudates. In (b) note the presence of active preretinal and intraretinal hemorrhage within the macula from bleeding neovascularization.

## Fluorescein angiography

FA should not be used routinely to screen patients with no or minimal diabetic retinopathy. FA is used as an adjunct to clinical examination to identify suspected but clinically obscure retinal neovascularization, which appears as areas of hyperfluorescence with late leakage (**Figure 2.3**). More commonly, FA is used as a guide for laser treatment in patients with clinically significant DME, as well as for evaluating the cause of unexplained vision loss such as macular ischemia.

## Red free photography

Red free images may demonstrate the presence of additional retinal hemorrhages, microaneurysms, and intraretinal microvascular abnormalities (IRMA) that may not be apparent on clinical examination.

## Ultrasonography

Ultrasonography is indicated to rule out retinal detachment in diabetic eyes with opaque media such as with dense cataract or vitreous hemorrhage.

# Further reading

Branch Vein Occlusion Study Group Argon laser photocoagulation for macular edema in branch vein occlusion. Am J Ophthalmol 1984; 98:271–82.

Brown DM, Campochiaro PA, Singh RP, et al. Ranibizumab for macular edema following central retinal vein occlusion: six-month primary end point results of a phase III study. Ophthalmology 2010; 117:1124–33.e1.

Brown DM, Heier JS, Clark WL, et al. Intravitreal aflibercept injection for macular edema secondary to central retinal vein occlusion: 1-year results for the phase 3 COPERNICUS study. Am J Ophthalmol 2013; 155:429–37.

Campochiaro PA, Heier JS, Feiner L, et al. Ranibizumab for macular edema following branch retinal vein occlusion: six-month primary end point results of a phase III study. Ophthalmology 2010; 117:1102–12.e1.

Central Vein Occlusion Study Group. Report: A randomized clinical trial of early panretinal photocoagulation for ischemic central vein occlusion. Ophthalmology 1995; 102:1434–44.

Central Vein Occlusion Study Group. Report: Evaluation of grid pattern photocoagulation for macular edema in central vein occlusion. Ophthalmology 1995; 102:1425–33.

Hayreh SS, Rojas P, Podhajsky P, Montague P, Woolson RF. Ocular neovascularization with retinal vascular occlusion-III. Incidence of ocular neovascularization with retinal vein occlusion. Ophthalmology 1983; 90:488–506.

Heier JS, Campochiaro PA, Yau L, et al. Ranibizumab for macular edema due to retinal vein occlusions: long-term follow-up in the HORIZON trial. Ophthalmology 2012; 119:802–9.

Ip MS, Scott IU, VanVeldhuisen PC, et al. A randomized trial comparing the efficacy and safety of intravitreal triamcinolone with observation to treat vision loss associated with macular edema secondary to central retinal vein occlusion: the Standard Care vs Corticosteroid for Retinal Vein Occlusion (SCORE) study report 5. Arch Ophthalmol 2009; 127:1101–14.

Jaulim A, Ahmed B, Khanam T, et al. Branch retinal vein occlusion: epidemiology, pathogenesis, risk factors, clinical features, diagnosis and complications: an update of the literature. Retina 2013; 33:901–10.

Central Vein Occlusion Study Group. Natural history and clinical management of central retinal vein occlusion. Arch Ophthalmol 1997; 115:486–91.

Eye Disease Case-control Study Group. Risk factors for branch retinal vein occlusion. Am J Ophthalmol 1993; 116:286–96.

Eye Disease Case-control Study Group. Risk factors for central retinal vein occlusion. Arch Ophthalmol 1996; 114:545–54.

Scott IU, Ip MS, VanVeldhuisen PC, et al. A randomized trial comparing the efficacy and safety of intravitreal triamcinolone with standard care to treat vision loss associated with macular Edema secondary to branch retinal vein occlusion: the Standard Care vs. Corticosteroid for Retinal Vein Occlusion (SCORE) study report 6. Arch Ophthalmol 2009; 127:1115–28.

Thach AB, Yau, L, Hoang C, Tuomi L. Time to clinically significant visual acuity gains after ranibizumab treatment for retinal vein occlusion: BRAVO and CRUISE trials. Ophthalmology 2014; 121:1059-66.

# Arterial occlusive disease

## How to approach a patient with vision loss and an acute occlusion of a retinal artery

| Identify the primary pathologic clinical finding(s) | | |
|---|---|---|
| On examination, the patient will demonstrate arterial occlusion with an area of retinal ischemia/whitening, and if acute, there may be the presence of a cherry-spot in the center of the macula. | | |
| **Formulate a differential diagnosis** | | |
| Most likely | Less likely | Least likely |
| • Central or branch retinal arterial obstruction | • Commotio retinae, infectious (herpetic) retinitis, ocular ischemic syndrome (OIS) | • Tay–Sachy's disease, Niemann–Pick's disease |
| **Query patient history** | | |
| • How long has the patient been experiencing symptoms?<br>• Any previous episodes of amaurosis fugax? Pain?<br>• Any history of trauma?<br>• Any previous history of stroke, atrial fibrillation, or carotid disease?<br>• Is the patient immunocompromised? | | |
| **Decide on ancillary diagnostic imaging** | | |
| The diagnosis of an arterial obstruction is clinically apparent acutely when there is diffuse retinal whitening secondary to ischemia in the territory of a retinal artery accompanied by abrupt, painless vision loss. Fluorescein angiography can be helpful for confirmation or in nonacute cases. | | |

## Ancillary diagnostic imaging interpretation

### Color fundus photographs

Color fundus photographs may demonstrate the presence of a cherry-red spot within the macula as well as retinal whitening and ischemia (**Figure 4.1**).

### Optical coherence tomography

Retinal thinning will be visible on optical coherence tomography in chronic cases with loss of the inner retina in areas of previous ischemia. Acutely, there may be retinal swelling in the region of ischemia (**Figure 4.2**).

### Fluorescein angiography

There is evidence of delayed arterial filling, often with a leading edge of dye in the region of the obstructed arteriole (**Figure 4.3**). Fluorescein angiography may also highlight emboli.

## Final diagnosis: retinal arteriole occlusion

### Epidemiology/etiology

Central retinal artery obstruction (CRAO) is rare, with the average patient age of 60 years. Men are affected twice as commonly as women.

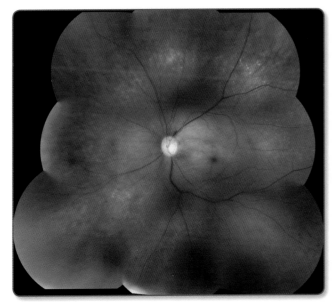

**Figure 4.1** Color mosaic photo of central retinal artery occlusion in the left eye. There is the classic cherry-red spot centrally with retinal whitening diffusely involving the macula. There is also a splinter hemorrhage in the peripapillary region.

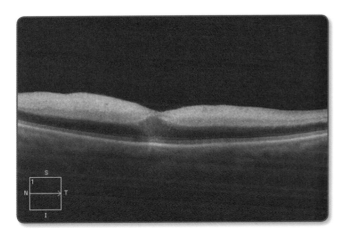

**Figure 4.2** Optical coherence tomography in new onset central retinal artery occlusion. Note the thickening of the inner retina consistent with swelling from acute infarction.

A central retinal arterial obstruction is most commonly due to thrombus formation at the region of the lamina cribrosa, the cause of which is most often related to atherosclerosis. Emboli are possible causes, but less common. Additional risk factors include hypercoagulable states, trauma, low-flow states from more proximal disease, optic disc drusen, active ocular infection, congenital abnormalities of the central retinal artery, and migraine. The presence of detectable emboli is visible in only 25% of patients.

Branch retinal artery obstruction (BRAO) more commonly affects the right eye and is more commonly related to emboli (two thirds of cases). Typically the emboli are visible at the arterial bifurcation, and originate from anywhere between the heart and ophthalmic artery.

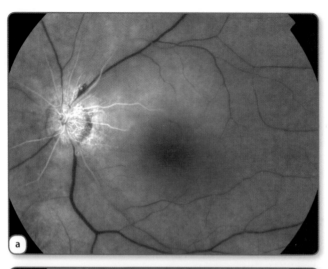

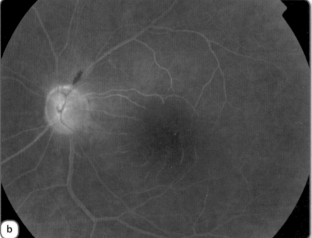

**Figure 4.3** Fluorescein angiogram of a central retinal artery occlusion in the left eye at 24 seconds (a) and 300 seconds (b). Note the leading edge of dye in the arteriole, which never completely fills.

Risk factors include hypertension, hypercholesterolemia, diabetes mellitus, smoking, and a positive family history.

## Symptoms and clinical findings

Patients with central artery occlusion present with painless, severe vision loss. Visual acuity is typically 20/800 or worse unless a cilioretinal artery is present and not involved. There is typically an afferent pupillary defect. On fundoscopy, there is retinal whitening indicative of acute ischemia. There may be the classic 'cherry-red' spot in the central macula that occurs because retinal ischemia causes blockage of the normal choroidal coloration everywhere except centrally where the nerve fiber layer is thin.

Associated features in central artery occlusion include previous episodes of amaurosis fugax, visible embolus in 25%, carotid artery disease in 33%, giant cell arteritis in 5%, neovascularization of the iris in 18%, and arterial collaterals on the optic disc.

Patients with branch retinal artery occlusion may present with sectoral visual field loss typically with preservation of central vision unless the cilioretinal artery is involved.

## Treatment/prognosis/follow-up

There is no proven treatment for central retinal artery occlusion. If central retinal artery obstruction is secondary to giant cell arteritis then treatment with high-dose corticosteroids is initiated to prevent contralateral vision loss.

Unfortunately, most central retinal arterial obstructions result in profound, permanent loss of vision. About one third of patients will experience some improvement in visual acuity. The patient should be worked up medically for causes of acute stroke and often these patients are admitted to the hospital for stroke evaluation. These patients can develop neovascularization of the retina, optic disc, and iris with subsequent neovascular glaucoma. Neovascularization is treated with the application of panretinal photocoagulation.

# Further reading

Arruga J, Sanders MD. Ophthalmologic findings in 70 patients with evidence of retinal embolism. Ophthalmology 1982; 89:1336–47.

Atebara NH, Brown GC, Cater J, et al. Efficacy of anterior chamber paracentesis and carbogen in treating nonarteritic central retinal artery obstruction. Ophthalmology 1995; 102:2029–35.

Brown GC, Magargal LE, Sergott R, et al. Acute obstruction of the retinal and choroidal circulations. Ophthalmology 1986; 93:1373–82.

Brown GC, Magargal LE. Central retinal artery obstruction and visual acuity. Ophthalmology 1982; 89:14–19.

Duker JS, Brown GC. Neovascularization of the optic disc associated with obstruction of the central retinal artery. Ophthalmology 1989; 96:87–91.

Duker JS, Brown GC. The efficacy of panretinal photocoagulation for neovascularization of the iris after central retinal artery obstruction. Ophthalmology 1989; 96:92–5.

Duker JS, Sivalingam A, Brown GC, et al. A prospective study of acute central retinal artery obstruction. Arch Ophthalmol 1991; 109:339–42.

Fineman MS, Savino PJ, Federman JL, et al. Branch retinal artery occlusion as the initial sign of giant cell arteritis. Am J Ophthalmol 1996; 112:428–30.

Hayreh SS, Podhajsky P. Ocular neovascularization with retinal vascular occlusion. Arch Ophthalmol 1982; 100:1585–96.

Sanborn GE, Magargal LE. Arterial obstructive disease of the eye. In: Tasman W, Jaeger EA (eds). Duane's Clinical Ophthalmology. Philadelphia, PA: Lippincott Williams & Wilkins; 2013.

# 5 Retinal arterial macroaneurysm

## How to approach a patient with a dilated, saccular arterial vessel

| Identify the primary pathologic clinical finding(s) | | |
|---|---|---|
| There is focal dilatation of a retinal artery within the first three orders of bifurcation. There are retinal hemorrhages that can be within all three layers of the retina including preretinal, intraretinal, and subretinal. There may be protein and lipid exudates along with macular edema. | | |
| **Formulate a differential diagnosis** | | |
| Most likely | Less likely | Least likely |
| • Retinal arterial macroaneurysm (RAM) | • Venous macroaneurysm, age-related macular degeneration, retinal capillary hemangioma, branch retinal vein obstruction | • Coat's disease, idiopathic juxtafoveal telegiectasia |
| **Query patient history** | | |
| • Does the patient have a history of hypertension?<br>• Has the patient previously had a retinal vein occlusion? | | |
| **Decide on ancillary diagnostic imaging** | | |
| The diagnosis of RAM is made clinically based on a characteristic fundus appearance with focal dilatation of a retinal artery within the first three orders of bifurcation. Diagnosis can be confirmed with fluorescein angiography (FA). Optical coherence tomography (OCT) is utilized to evaluate for the presence of macular edema. RAM is one of the few entities that can cause simultaneous subretinal, intraretinal, and preretinal hemorrhage. | | |

## Ancillary diagnostic imaging interpretation

### Color photography

Color fundus photography is not required for the diagnosis of RAM, but can be used to demonstrate the presence of a focal dilated retinal artery, retinal hemorrhages, lipid exudation, and the presence of macular edema (**Figure 5.1**).

### Optical coherence tomography

OCT is helpful in determining if there is associated macular edema, lipid exudates within the fovea that may limit visual recovery, and in monitoring response to therapy (**Figure 5.2**).

### Fluorescein angiography

FA can confirm the presence of RAM. There is immediate complete filling of the macroaneurysm; however, if there is partial thrombosis there may be incomplete filling. In active lesions, there may be associated leakage from the wall of the aneurysm (**Figure 5.3**).

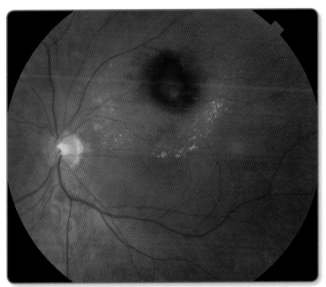

**Figure 5.1** Color fundus photograph demonstrating a typical retinal arterial macroaneurysm. Note the presence of preretinal and intraretinal hemorrhage surrounding a dilated focal outpouching of a retinal vessel. This is associated with a circinate ring of hard exudates.

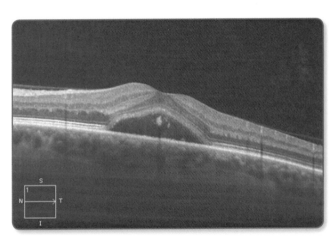

**Figure 5.2** Optical coherence tomography through the fovea (corresponding to Figure 5.1) in a patient with a retinal arterial macroaneurysm. Note the presence of subretinal fluid and hard exudates beneath the fovea.

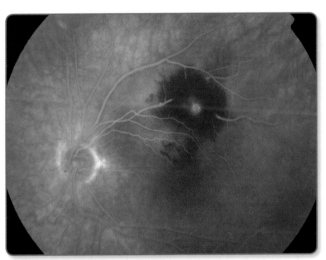

**Figure 5.3** Fluorescein angiogram, late frame (corresponding to Figure 5.1) in a patient with a retinal arterial macroaneurysm. Note the dilated macroaneurysm that appears to be leaking as well as the blockage from retinal hemorrhage (both preretinal and intraretinal).

## Indocyanine green angiography

When there is dense retinal hemorrhage RAM may not be visible on FA. In this case, indocyanine green angiography can be a helpful adjunct tool for diagnosis. Because the absorption and emission spectrum is near infrared range, the dye can penetrate more easily through hemorrhage.

# Final diagnosis: retinal arterial macroaneurysm

## Epidemiology/etiology

RAM more commonly occurs in patients over 60 years of age and is more common in women. It is typically unilateral although may be bilateral in 10% of cases and multifocal in some. RAM is associated with systemic hypertension; however, the exact pathogenesis is not completely understood. There is also an association with branch retinal vein occlusion. Saccular or 'blowout aneuryms' are more likely to bleed and more classically arise closer to the optic nerve head because of higher perfusion pressures. Fusiform dilations are more likely to result in lipid exudation and are more commonly associated with a history of venous occlusion.

## Symptoms and clinical findings

RAM has a variable presentation. It may be an incidental finding and asymptomatic. If associated with macular edema or vitreous hemorrhage then there is associated visual compromise. Submacular hemorrhage may be toxic to the retina and the formation of fibrin clot can cause permanent structural damage resulting in vision loss centrally.

## Treatment/prognosis/follow-up

Historical treatments for RAM include using the xenon arc, argon, and yellow dye laser both directly at and around the macroaneurysm; however, there have been no large prospective trials proving the efficacy of ablative treatment, and several small case series demonstrating mixed results.

In general, hemorrhagic macroaneurysms tends to have a better prognosis than exudative macroaneurysms in terms of final visual acuity. The hemorrhagic macroaneurysms tend to thrombose and the retinal and vitreous hemorrhage clear. Because of this, these patients are often observed for a few months. Patients with exudative macroaneurysms often have worse outcomes, and therefore laser treatment is more often considered for treatment. When laser is performed it is with yellow dye laser or argon green with large spot size >500 mm in diameter and longer burn duration of 0.2–0.5 seconds.

Additional laser treatments have been tried to treat premacular and submacular hemorrhage associated with RAM. Neodymium:yttrium-aluminum-garnet (Nd:YAG) laser has been tried for dense premacular hemorrhage to speed visual recovery and possibly limit macular detachment. The goal of this laser treatment is to disrupt the hyaloid face and allow for drainage of the blood into the vitreous cavity. There are some studies that demonstrate more rapid visual recovery using this technique; however, complications such as vitreous hemorrhage, macular hole, and retinal detachment have been described. Additional therapies such as pneumatic displacement with or without the use of intravitreal tissue plasminogen activator for submacular hemorrhage have been tried with variable success.

# Further reading

Abdel-Khalek MN, Richardson J. Retinal macroaneurysm: natural history and guidelines for treatment. Br J Ophthalmol 1986; 70:2–11.

Asdourian GK, Goldberg MF, Jampol LM, et al. Retinal macroaneurysms. Arch Ophthalmol 1977; 95:624–8.

Hassan AS, Johnson MW, Schneiderman TE, et al. Management of submacular hemorrhage with intravitreous tissue plasminogen activator injection and pneumatic displacement. Ophthalmology 1999; 106:1900–1907.

Mainster MA, Whitacre MM. Dye yellow photocoagulation of retinal arterial macroaneurysms. Am J Ophthalmol 1988; 105:97–8.

McCabe CM, Flynn HW, McLean WC, et al. Nonsurgical management of macular hemorrhage secondary to retinal artery macroaneurysms. Arch Ophthalmol 2000; 118:780–85.

Nadel AJ, Gupta KK. Macroaneurysms of the retinal arteries. Arch Ophthalmol 1976;94:1092–6.

Palestine AG, Robertson DM, Goldstein BG, et al. Macroaneurysms of the retinal arteries. Am J Ophthalmol 1982; 93:164–71.

Panton RW, Goldberg MF, Farber MD, et al. Retinal arterial macroaneurysms: risk factors and natural history. Br J Ophthalmol 1990; 74:595–600.

Robertson DM. Macroaneurysms of the retinal arteries. Trans Am Acad Ophthalmol Otolaryngol 1973;77.

Russel SR, Folk JC. Branch retinal artery occlusion after dye yellow photocoagulation of an arterial macroaneurysm. Am J Ophthalmol. 1987; 104:186–7.

Townsend-Pico WA, Meyers SM, Lewis H, et al. Indocyanine green angiography in the diagnosis of retinal arterial macroaneurysms associated with submacular and preretinal hemorrhages: a case series. Am J Ophthalmol 2000; 129:33–7.

## How to approach a patient with retinal hemorrhages, cotton-wool spots, and a history of head/neck radiation

| Identify the primary pathologic clinical finding(s) | | |
|---|---|---|
| There may be retinal microaneurysms, hemorrhages, telangiectatic vessels, hard exudates, macular edema, cotton wool spots or optic disc swelling. Neovascularization of both the anterior and posterior segment can be seen. These clinical signs may be singular or multiple depending on the severity. | | |
| **Formulate a differential diagnosis** | | |
| **Most likely** | **Less likely** | **Least likely** |
| • Radiation retinopathy | • Diabetic retinopathy, hypertensive retinopathy, retinal venous occlusion, HIV retinopathy | • Leukemia, coagulopathy, Coats' disease, juxtafoveal telangiectasia, ischemic optic neuropathy, optic neuritis, papilledema |
| **Query patient history** | | |
| • Any history of previous head or neck radiation or cancer?<br>• Does the patient have diabetes, hypertension, or collagen vascular disease?<br>• Any pain with eye movement, headaches, or trouble with color vision? | | |
| **Decide on ancillary diagnostic imaging** | | |
| Radiation retinopathy is a clinical diagnosis that is made when there are signs of ischemic retinopathy or papillopathy and a history of previous ionizing radiation. Optical coherence tomography (OCT) may be used to demonstrate the presence of macular edema. Fluorescein angiography (FA) can be used to demonstrate areas of retinal ischemia. | | |

## Ancillary diagnostic imaging interpretation

### Color fundus photography

Color fundus photography may be used for exam documentation, but is not necessary. There may be many or few signs including retinal hemorrhages, cotton-wool spots, macular edema, and hard exudates (**Figure 6.1**).

### Optical coherence tomography

OCT is useful to demonstrate the presence of macular edema as well as monitor response to treatment (**Figure 6.2**).

### Fluorescein angiography

FA can be used to demonstrate capillary dropout and areas of retinal ischemia as well as the presence of macular edema, optic nerve edema, and neovascularization.

## Final diagnosis: radiation retinopathy

### Epidemiology/etiology

The risk of radiation retinopathy is determined by the total dose of radiation administered to the retina, as well as the fraction size of the

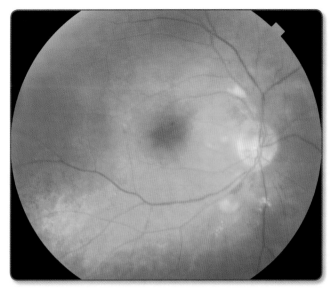

**Figure 6.1** Color fundus photograph of the right eye demonstrating radiation retinopathy. Note the presence of multiple retinal hemorrhages within the macula as well as peripapillary region, cotton-wool spots, and hard exudates. There is decreased foveal light reflex that likely reflects underlying macular edema.

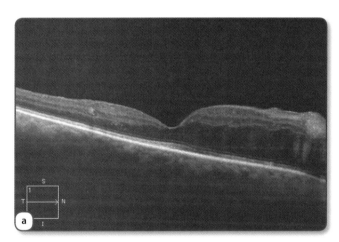

**Figure 6.2** Optical coherence tomography of the macula (a) including both the five lines and macular cube (b) demonstrating macular edema from the eye in Figure 6.1, which appears to be originating from the optic nerve.

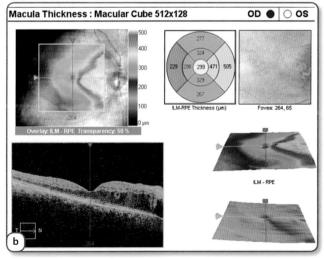

radiation. Brachytherapy for choroidal melanoma within 5 mm of the macula carries a significant risk. The risk increases with doses of radiation >4500 rad (45 Gy). Patients who receive radiation <2500 rad (25 Gy) in doses <200 rad (2 Gy) are at relatively low risk.

The exact incidence of radiation retinopathy is unknown; however, around 50% of patients treated for orbital, nasopharyngeal, or paranasal neoplasms will develop some retinopathy. The time course is typically 2–3 years after exposure. Patients with a history of diabetes, hypertension, collagen vascular disease, leukemia, or undergoing chemotherapy are at additional risk.

Ionizing radiation causes damage to the inner retina, primarily affecting the retinal nerve fiber layer, while preserving the outer retina. There is loss of vascular endothelial cells that leads to nonperfusion, ischemia, and ultimately neuronal degeneration and gliosis.

With more intense radiation over 60 Gy, there can also be direct toxicity to the retinal photoreceptors, choriocapillaries, retinal pigment epithelial cells, inner retina, and optic nerve.

## Symptoms and clinical findings

Small amounts of retinopathy may be asymptomatic. The presence of dilated telangiectatic channels at the macula without a significant number of microaneurysms, venous beading, or evidence of neovascularization is consistent with radiation retinopathy.

Symptoms develop with the presence of macular edema, optic nerve papillopathy, or neovascularization. Radiation optic neuropathy can appear clinically similar to anterior ischemic optic neuropathy but more commonly occurs in younger patients without a history of hypertension, with the notable absence of involvement of the posterior ciliary vessels on angiography.

## Treatment/prognosis/follow-up

There is no treatment necessary for mild retinopathy that is not impacting vision. These patients, however, should be followed frequently as the retinopathy may be progressive. Patients with nonproliferative retinopathy on average retain a visual acuity of 20/50 for at least 4 years.

There are no randomized controlled clinical trials of treatment for radiation retinopathy. For macular edema, similarly to patients with diabetic retinopathy, focal or grid laser can be utilized. Additionally, anti-VEGF therapy and intravitreal corticosteroids may be tried; however, these are considered off-label usage and unproven by clinical trial. There has been some recent evidence that anti-VEGF treatment within the first year after radiation therapy for ocular melanoma may decrease the risk of development of significant retinopathy. Neovascularization, as with all causes of ischemic retinopathy, is treated with panretinal photocoagulation. Patients with proliferative retinopathy have a much worse visual prognosis, with the majority retaining vision of <20/200 after 6 years.

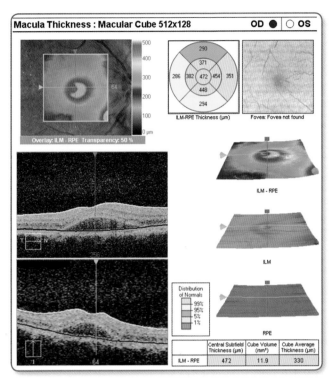

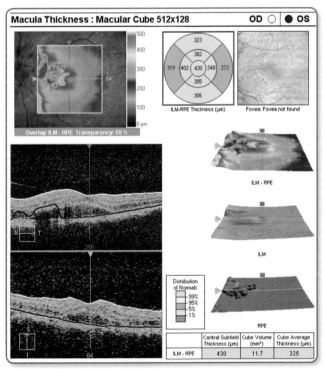

**Figure 7.3** Optical coherence tomography of the macula in a patient with malignant hypertension. Note the presence of bilateral subretinal fluid through the fovea.

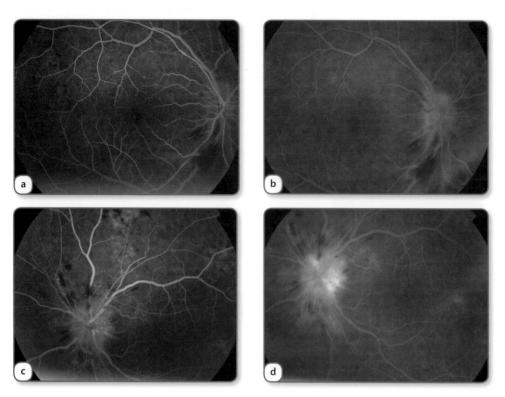

**Figure 7.4** Fluorescein angiography in a patient with malignant hypertension with early and late images of the left eye (a, b) and right eye (c, d). Note the presence of bilateral early blockage from retinal hemorrhage and late leakage around the optic nerve consistent with edema.

## Treatment/prognosis/follow-up

Patients with asymptomatic hypertensive retinopathy require no treatment but should be followed annually with a dilated eye examination. These patients should also be advised that blood pressure control is important to prevent the progression of retinopathy as well as for their overall health.

Patients with acute hypertensive crisis and vision loss need to be identified, and followed closely with comanagement of the hypertension with an internist. The mortality rate for untreated malignant hypertension is 50% at 2 months and 90% at 1 year. There is no ophthalmic treatment for this disease other than medically controlling the blood pressure. Prognosis for visual recovery is excellent with most patients retaining good vision. Vision loss can occur from optic nerve atrophy secondary to prolonged edema, or retinal changes from chronic macular edema.

# Further reading

Hayreh SS, Servais GE, Vridi PS. Fundus lesions in malignant hypertension. IV. Focal intraretinal periarteriolar transudates. Ophthalmology. 1986; 93:60–73.

Keith NM, Wagener HP, Barker NW. Some different types of essential hypertension: their course and prognosis. Am J Med Sci 1939; 197:332–43.

Kincaid-Smith P, McMichael J, Murphy EA. The clinical course and pathology of hypertension with papilloedema (malignant hypertension). Q J Med 1958; 27:117–53.

Klein R, Kelin BE, Moss SE, et al. Hypertension and retinopathy, arteriolar narrowing, and arteriovenous nicking in a population. Arch Ophthalmol. 1994; 112:92–8.

# Sickle cell retinopathy

## How to approach a patient with peripheral nonperfusion and neovascularization

| Identify the primary pathologic clinical finding(s) | | |
|---|---|---|
| There may be evidence of salmon patches, black sunbursts, peripheral nonperfusion, 'sea-fan' neovascularization, and macular ischemia. | | |
| **Formulate a differential diagnosis** | | |
| **Most likely** | **Less likely** | **Least likely** |
| • Sickle cell retinopathy, proliferative diabetic retinopathy, branch retinal vein obstruction | • Ocular ischemic syndrome, sarcoidosis, retinopathy of prematurity, chronic retinal detachment, retinal vasculitis, pars planitis | • Retinopathy of prematurity, Eales' disease, familial exudative vitreoretinopathy |
| **Query patient history** | | |
| • Does the patient have a history of sickle cell disease or trait personally or within the family? <br> • Does the patient have a history of diabetes? <br> • Was the patient born premature? <br> • Does the patient have a history of previous intraocular infection? <br> • Does the patient have a history of autoimmune disease, stroke, or carotid artery disease? | | |
| **Decide on ancillary diagnostic imaging** | | |
| Color wide field imaging allows for documentation of peripheral retinal abnormalities but is not required for diagnosis (**Figure 8.1**). Wide field angiography or fluorescein angiography (FA) with peripheral sweeps is useful for evaluating peripheral vascular abnormalities. Optical coherence tomography (OCT) can be utilized to evaluate for the presence of macular ischemia although is not used routinely in screening asymptomatic patients. | | |

## Ancillary diagnostic imaging interpretation

### Optical coherence tomography

OCT may demonstrate the presence of macular ischemia with loss of the outer retina secondary to previous infarction.

### Fluorescein angiography

FA with peripheral sweeps or wide field angiography can be used to demonstrate the presence of peripheral nonperfusion as well as for demonstrating the presence of 'sea-fan' neovascularization, macular edema or macular ischemia, as well as more subtle arterial or venous changes (**Figure 8.2**).

## Final diagnosis: sickle cell retinopathy

### Epidemiology/etiology

Normal hemoglobin is made up of two alpha and two beta chains and is referred to as hemoglobin A. Sickle hemoglobin, known as hemoglobin S, has a mutation such that the amino acid valine is substituted for glutamic acid. Hemoglobin C occurs with the substitution of lysine

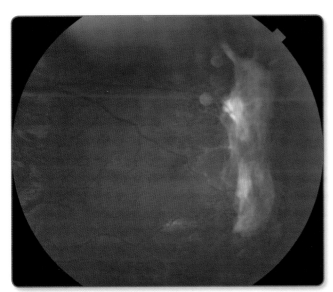

**Figure 8.1** Color fundus photograph of the retinal periphery demonstrating 'sea-fan' neovascularization in sickle cell retinopathy. Note the active fibrovascular proliferation on top of the neovascularization.

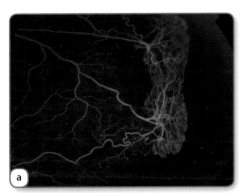

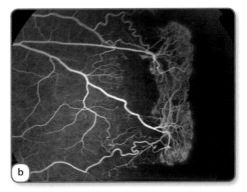

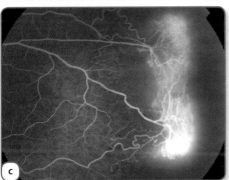

**Figure 8.2** (a) Early-, (b) mid-, and (c) late-frame fluorescein angiogram of peripheral 'sea-fan' neovascularization in sickle cell retinopathy. Note the peripheral ischemia as well as the late leakage of fluorescein consistent with active neovascularization.

for glutamic acid. Thalassemia occurs when there is inadequate production of hemoglobin.

Normal hemoglobin is pliable and allows the red blood cells to easily pass through the microvasculature throughout the body. In sickle cell hemoglobin, the red blood cells assume an abnormal shape, particularly under conditions of acidity or hypoxia, causing the red blood cells to stack up causing ischemia. This in turn leads to a cycle of sickling, tissue hypoxia, and necrosis.

In the United States, African Americans account for the majority of patients with sickle cell disease, sickle cell trait, and thalassemia. In African Americans, the prevalence of sickle trait is 5–10%. From a systemic perspective, full sickle cell disease (SS) is most severe; however, hemoglobin S-Thal and hemoglobin SC disease result in more severe ophthalmic disease. This may be related to the fact that in full sickle cell disease there is greater anemia, which may mean there are less red blood cells overall to get lodged in the microvasculature of the retina.

## Symptoms and clinical findings

Anterior segment symptoms include comma-shaped capillaries that occur because of intravascular sludging of red blood cells. There can also be mild anterior chamber cell and flare and the presence of synechiae because of disruption of the blood/ocular barrier. These anterior chamber findings are usually asymptomatic.

Sickle cell retinopathy has both nonproliferative and proliferative changes. Venous tortuosity is seen in about 50% of patients with SS disease and 33% patients with sickle cell disease but is nonspecific. More characteristic changes include a 'salmon patch,' which is a preretinal or superficial intraretinal hemorrhage that occurs adjacent to a retinal arteriole, often at the equator. Initially these lesions are bright red but turn more pink over time and are due to rupture of a medium-size retinal arteriole secondary to ischemia. These lesions usually resolve without complication; however, sometimes a retinoschisis cavity may persist. Also characteristic is a 'black sunburst' lesion that occurs if the intraretinal hemorrhage disturbs the retinal pigment epithelium causing retinal pigment epithelial hyperplasia and intraretinal migration. These lesions are also asymptomatic (**Figure 8.3**).

Proliferative sickle cell retinopathy may cause vision loss and has been divided into five stages. The first stage is peripheral arteriolar occlusion, which leads to peripheral nonperfusion. The second stage is arteriolar-venous anastomoses, which is seen at the junction of perfused and nonperfused retina. The third stage is neovascular proliferation; the classic sign appears in a 'sea-fan' configuration (**Figure 8.1**). The fourth stage is vitreous hemorrhage, which can occur spontaneously or secondary to mild ocular trauma. The fifth stage is retinal detachment, which develops secondary to fibrovascular proliferation along the areas of neovascularization.

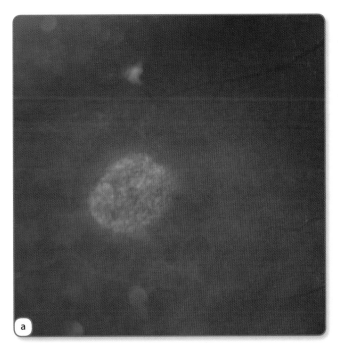

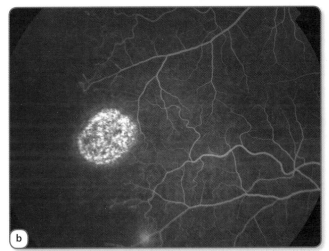

**Figure 8.3** Color fundus photograph (a) and corresponding fluorescein angiography (b) of peripheral retinal sunburst from a patient with sickle cell retinopathy. Note the peripheral nonperfusion temporal to the lesion.

## Treatment/prognosis/follow-up

There is no known treatment to reduce the risk of progression of sickle cell retinopathy despite our understanding of the disease pathogenesis. Treatment is reserved for proliferative sickle cell retinopathy to reduce the risk of progression to vitreous hemorrhage or retinal detachment. Scatter peripheral retinal laser photocoagulation is performed either to areas of nonperfused retina or to the full peripheral retina. Other modalities such as cryotherapy and diathermy have been abandoned because of the higher complication rates. Vitreous hemorrhage from proliferative sickle cell retinopathy may be observed for 3–6 months, prior to vitrectomy with endolaser if the hemorrhage persists. Tractional retinal detachments are treated if macula involving or macula threatening. It is important to note that patients with sickle hemoglobinopathies are at higher risk for thromboembolic events during surgery. Additionally, preoperative ocular risks include anterior segment ischemia, optic nerve, and macular infarcts, which can occur with intraocular pressures as low as 25 mmHg.

Patients with nonproliferative sickle cell retinopathy are generally free from any visual complaints and should be followed yearly. The prognosis of patients with proliferative sickle cell retinopathy is highly variable. Untreated the risk of blindness is about 12%. Patients with proliferative retinopathy need to be followed closely until stabilized.

# Further reading

Goldberg MF. Classification and pathogenesis of proliferative sickle retinopathy. Am J Ophthalmol 1971; 71:649–65.

Goldberg MF. Natural history of untreated proliferative sickle retinopathy. Arch Ophthalmol 1971; 72:35–50.

Romayananda N, Goldberg MF, Green WR. Histopathology of sickle cell retinopathy. Trans Am Acad Ophthalmol Otolaryngol 1973; 77:642–76.

Van Meurs JC. Evolution of a retinal hemorrhage in a patient with sickle cell-hemoglobin C disease. Arch Ophthalmol 1995; 113:1074–5.

# Macular telangiectasia and Coats' disease

## How to approach a patient with retinal telangiectasias and hard exudates

| Identify the primary pathologic clinical finding(s) | | |
|---|---|---|
| There is abnormal development of retinal vasculature, characterized by retinal telangiectasias and intraretinal and subretinal exudate. There may be associated serous retinal detachment in severe cases. | | |
| **Formulate a differential diagnosis** | | |
| Most likely | Less likely | Least likely |
| • Coats' disease, macular telangiectasia (type 1), familial exudative vitreoretinopathy, retinopathy of prematurity | • Ocular toxocariasis, retinal capillary hemangioma, retinoblastoma | • Persistent fetal vasculature, incontinentia pigmenti (IP, Bloch–Sulzberger syndrome), Norrie disease, pars planitis |
| **Query patient history** | | |
| • Is there a family history of retinal detachment or blindness/retinopathy?<br>• Was the patient born prematurely?<br>• Did the patient receive oxygen therapy?<br>• Are there any congenital or systemic abnormalities?<br>• Does the patient have any hearing loss or muscle weakness? | | |
| **Decide on ancillary diagnostic imaging** | | |
| Coats' disease is diagnosed clinically with indirect ophthalmoscopic identification of retinovascular abnormalities and intraretinal and/or subretinal exudate. Fluorescein angiography is helpful to further characterize retinovascular abnormalities. B-scan ultrasonography, CT scan, and MRI may also be required to rule out imitators such as retinoblastoma. | | |

## Ancillary diagnostic imaging interpretation

### Color fundus photography

Color fundus photographs are useful to document the extent of disease, monitor for new lesions, and assess response to therapy (**Figure 10.1**).

### Optical coherence tomography

Optical coherence tomography is useful to evaluate for the presence of macular edema and subretinal fluid, as well as to monitor response to therapy (**Figure 10.2**).

### Fluorescein angiography

Fluorescein angiography is the key for diagnosis and for assessing response to therapy. It enables visualization of the characteristic vascular changes, which may be remotely located from the area of retinal exudate. Observed features include retinal vascular telangiectasias, aneurysmal dilations, which are often referred to as 'light bulb' aneurysms, venous beading and sheathing and areas of nonperfusion (**Figure 10.3**). Telangiectasias show early hyperfluorescence with late leakage, while exudates blocks fluorescence.

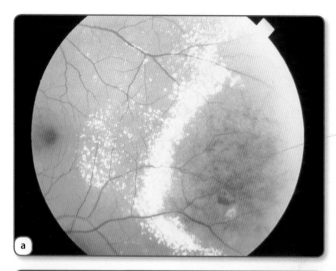

a

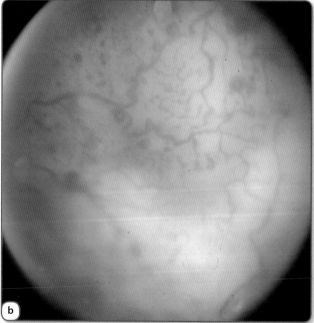

b

**Figure 10.1** (a) Stage 2 Coats' disease demonstrating abnormal retinal vasculature surrounded by exudate temporal to the fovea. (b) Color fundus photograph demonstrates typical retinovascular abnormalities and subretinal exudate in Coats' disease.

## B-scan ultrasonography

In eyes with exudative retinal detachment, B-scan can be useful to evaluate for the presence of a subretinal mass, as well as characterize the type of subretinal fluid.

## CT scan and MRI

CT scan may be helpful for atypical cases to evaluate for the presence of a solitary tumor, calcification, extraocular extension, or neurologic

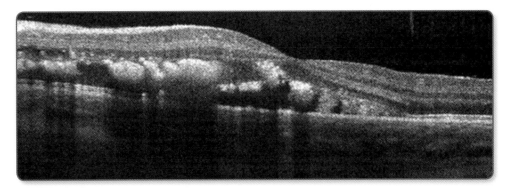

**Figure 10.2** Optical coherence tomography in a patient with Coats' disease. Note the presence of hard exudates underneath the fovea associated with subretinal fluid.

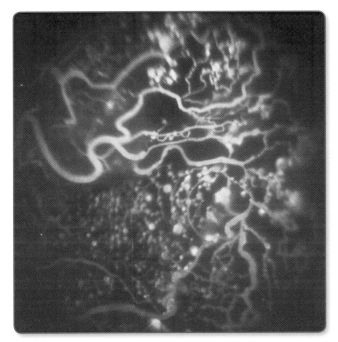

**Figure 10.3** Fluorescein angiogram in a patient with Coats' disease reveals telangiectasia, aneurysmal dilations, and peripheral capillary nonperfusion.

involvement, which may be seen with retinoblastoma, as well as to exclude other imitators.

# Final diagnosis: Coats' disease

## Epidemiology/etiology

Coats' disease, also known as retinal telangiectasia, is a rare, idiopathic disorder characterized by defective retinal vascular development. It occurs in males in over 85% of cases. It is described as unilateral in the majority of cases although fluorescein angiographic studies have demonstrated a higher rate of bilateral vascular abnormalities than previously thought. It is usually diagnosed in childhood between ages 8 and 16 years; however, adult onset can occur. Typically adult onset cases are less severe at presentation, and have a more limited area of retinal involvement, and slower progression. Coats' disease has traditionally been described as idiopathic and nonhereditary; however, more recent work suggests that there may also be a genetic component. Somatic mutation in the NDP gene, which encodes a protein norrin thought to be important for normal vascular development, may be abnormal in both Coats' and Norrie disease.

Retinal telangiectasia identical to Coats' disease has been described in association with other disorders but is extremely rare. The most notable is retinal telangiectasia as an extramuscular manifestation of facioscapulohumeral muscular dystrophy. This finding is usually bilateral, occurs more commonly in females, and is associated with sensorineural hearing loss. When retinal telangiectasia and exudate develop due to another disease, this is termed Coats' response and has been described secondary to retinitis pigmentosa.

## Symptoms and clinical findings

One quarter of cases of Coats' disease are discovered in asymptomatic patients during routine examination. Coats' disease can also present with decreased vision related to macular edema, leukocoria due to subretinal exudate or exudative detachment or elevated intraocular pressure or eye pain from neovascular glaucoma. When the disease presents in childhood, it is usually more severe. The anterior segment is usually unaffected in early stages of Coats' disease. In advanced stages, there may be iris and angle neovascularization, signs of anterior segment ischemia with cataract or cholesterol crystals in the anterior chamber. Anterior segment findings indicate severe disease with a less favorable prognosis. Cells in the vitreous or anterior chamber are usually not associated with Coats' disease and if present, another etiology should be considered.

Clinical features that may assist differentiation of Coats' disease from retinoblastoma including the color of pupillary light reflex and subretinal fluid (yellow in Coats', white gray in retinoblastoma), nature of the retinal blood vessels that are irregular with aneurysms and remain visible in Coats' disease and are regular in size and disappear into the tumor in retinoblastoma and the presence or absence of a solitary mass with imaging (CT, ultrasound, MRI).

A classification of Coats' disease as proposed by Shields and coauthors is outlined in **Table 10.1**. The earliest stage (stage 1) is the development of a localized area of retinal telangiectasia and aneurysmal dilations. These are more often fusiform and referred to as light bulb aneurysms. Venous dilation, sheathing, and areas of capillary nonperfusion may be present. These changes are often noted temporally or inferiorly at the equatorial and peripheral retina. This

| Table 10.1 Staging and vision in Coats' disease | | | |
|---|---|---|---|
| Stage, severity | Clinical finding | Vision <20/200 | Treatment options |
| 1, Mild | Retinal telangiectasia/aneurysms only | Rare | Laser photocoagulation, cryotherapy, observation |
| 2A, Mild | Telangiectasia and exudate (extrafoveal) | 50% | Laser photocoagulation, cryotherapy |
| 2B | Telangiectasia and exudate (foveal) | | Laser photocoagulation, cryotherapy, adjuvant therapy |
| 3A, Advanced | Subtotal exudative retinal detachment | 75% | Laser photocoagulation, adjuvant therapy, cryotherapy |
| 3B | Total exudative retinal detachment | | Vitreoretinal surgery, adjuvant therapy, cryotherapy, observation |
| 4 | Total detachment and secondary glaucoma | 100% | Observation, enucleation |
| 5 | End stage (prephthisical) | 100% | Observation, enucleation |

Modified from Shields et al. (2000).
Adjuvant therapy is intravitreal injection with triamcinolone or VEGF inhibitor.

can lead to retinovascular leakage with intraretinal and subretinal exudation (stage 2). Over time without treatment, this may slowly progresses to exudative retinal detachment (stage 3), onto neovascular glaucoma (stage 4), and prephthisis bulbi (stage 5).

## Treatment/prognosis/follow-up

There are several treatment options available, and the modality depends on the stage as outlined in **Table 10.1**. The aim of therapy is to ablate the abnormal retina vessels in order to prevent progression to retinal detachment and preserve vision and anatomy. Peripheral scatter laser and cryotherapy are used for mild-to-moderate disease and may be used combined with another modality such as surgery for advanced disease. Laser photocoagulation is used to cauterize the abnormal vessels and to treat avascular peripheral retina. Multiple sessions of laser are often necessary. Laser is typically most useful in attached retina, as it may not be able to penetrate through thick exudate to reach the underlying aberrant vessels. Cryotherapy may be useful when exudative disease is present, and like with laser, multiple sessions may be needed. However, excessive cryotherapy may increase subretinal exudation and retinal detachment; therefore, it has been recommended to treat only two quadrants of retina per session and wait at least a month between treatments.

Intravitreal injections may be used combined with other treatments. Intravitreal triamcinolone has been reported to improve macular exudate and edema. Anti-VEGF agents, primarily bevacizumab, but also ranibizumab and pegaptanib, have been used with reported success in small series. Photodynamic therapy combined with bevacizumab has also been utilized. Surgery may be considered in selected eyes with total exudative retinal detachment. Enucleation may be considered for a painful eye with neovascular glaucoma and total exudative retinal detachment that lacks visual potential.

# Further reading

Beby F, Roche O, Burillon C, Denis P. Coats' disease and bilateral cataract in a child with Turner syndrome: a case report. Graefes Arch Clin Exp Ophthalmol 2005; 243:1291–93.

Black GCM, Perveen R, Bonshek R, et al. Coats' disease of the retina (unilateral retinal telangiectasis) caused by somatic mutation in the NDP gene: a role for norrin in retinal angiogenesis. Hum Mol Genet 1999; 8:2031–5.

Dickinson JL, Sale MM, Passmore A, et al. Mutations in the NDP gene: contribution to Norrie disease, familial exudative vitreoretinopathy ad retinopathy of prematurity. Clin Exp Ophthalmol 2006; 34:682–8.

Henry CR, Berrocal AM, Hess DJ, Murray TG. Intraoperative spectral-domain optical coherence tomography in Coats' disease. Ophthalmic Surg Lasers Imaging 2012; 43:e80–84

Kase S, Rao NA, Yoshikawa H, et al. Expression of vascular endothelial growth factor in eyes with Coats' disease. Invest Ophthalmol Vis Sci 2013; 54:57–62.

Newell SW, Hall BD, Anderson CW, Lim ES. Hallermann-Streiff syndrome with Coats' disease. J Pediatr Ophthalmol Strabismus 1994; 31:123–5.

Schuman JS, Lieberman KV, Friedman AH, et al. Senior-Loken syndrome (familial renal-retinal dystrophy) and Coats' disease. Am J Ophthalmol 1985; 100:822–7.

Shields JA, Shields CL, Honavar SG, Demirci H. Clinical variations and complications of Coats' disease in 150 cases: the 2000 Sanford Gifford Memorial Lecture. Am J Ophthalmol 2001; 131:561–71.

Shields JA, Shields CL, Honavar SG, Demirci H, Cater J. Classification and management of Coats disease: the 2000 Proctor Lecture. Am J Ophthalmol 2001; 131:572–83.

Smithen LM, Brown GC, Brucker AJ, et al. Coats' disease diagnosed in adulthood. Ophthalmology 2005; 112:1072–8.

# 12

# Dry age-related macular degeneration

## How to approach a patient with drusen and retinal pigment epithelial changes

| Identify the primary pathologic clinical finding(s) | | |
|---|---|---|
| There are bilateral drusen, retinal pigment epithelial changes, and possible pigment epithelial detachment and geographic atrophy. | | |
| **Formulate a differential diagnosis** | | |
| Most likely | Less likely | Least likely |
| • Dry age-related macular degeneration, neovascular age-related macular degeneration | • Pattern dystrophy, adult onset vitelliform dystrophy, Stargardt's disease | • Toxic maculopathy (e.g. Plaquenil), multifocal choroiditis, macular telangiectasias type II, maternally inherited diabetes and deafness |
| **Query patient history** | | |
| • Is there a family history of age-related macular degeneration (ARMD) or early onset vision loss? <br> • Any recent change in vision? <br> • Any previous history of intravitreal injections? <br> • Any medication use? <br> • Does the patient smoke cigarettes? | | |
| **Decide on ancillary diagnostic imaging** | | |
| Macular degeneration is diagnosed with clinical examination of the macula. Fundus photography, fundus autofluorescence (FAF), optical coherence tomography (OCT), and fluorescein angiography (FA) can be used for further assessment. | | |

## Ancillary diagnostic imaging interpretation

### Color fundus photography

Color fundus (CF) photography is useful to document the presence of drusen, retinal pigment epithelial (RPE) disturbances as well as areas of geographic atrophy (**Figures 12.1** and **12.2**). CF photography is used in ARMD studies for grading purposes and can be used clinically to follow the progression of the disease over time.

### Optical coherence tomography

OCT is the main tool used to evaluate patients with macular degeneration. Drusen can be visualized as small deposits underneath Bruch's membrane. Geographic atrophy is also visualized on OCT with absence of the outer layers of the retina (**Figures 12.3** and **12.4**). The absence of subretinal or intraretinal fluid is important to rule out conversion to neovascular age-related macular degeneration.

### Fluorescein angiography

FA is used to evaluate for the presence of choroidal neovascularization. In dry ARMD, there is notable absence of any late leakage (**Figure 12.5**).

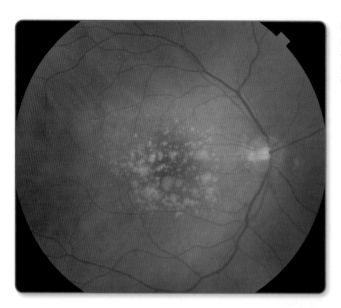

**Figure 12.1** Color fundus photograph of the right eye in a patient with dry age-related macular degeneration. Note the extensive drusen.

## Fundus autofluorescence

FAF may highlight areas of sick or atrophic retinal pigment epithelium (hypo autofluorescence) as well as demonstrate the presence of drusen that appear hyper autofluorescent (**Figure 12.6**). Areas of geographic atrophy demonstrate very low to extinguished FAF due to the loss of RPE and lipofuscin.

## Final diagnosis: dry age-related macular degeneration

### Epidemiology/etiology

The WHO estimated that in 2002, 14 million patients were blind or severely visually impaired from age-related macular degeneration, and it is a leading cause of vision loss among patients over 65 years of age in developed countries. The prevalence varies according to gender and race, and Caucasian females are at higher risk. Other risks factors include advancing age, smoking, obesity, and family history.

The exact pathogenesis of ARMD has not been fully elucidated; early in the course of the disease, lipids are deposited underneath Bruch's membrane, which occurs prior to the formation of visible drusen. There is concurrent thickening of Bruch's membrane, degeneration of elastin and collagen within Bruch's membrane, calcification, and accumulation of exogenous proteins and lipids. There is activation of the complement cascade that ultimately causes damage to retinal photoreceptors and vision loss.

### Symptoms and clinical findings

Drusen are usually the earliest clinical finding in ARMD. Most commonly they are found in the posterior pole but they can occur

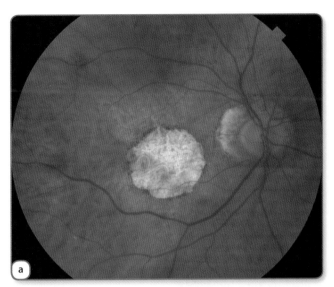

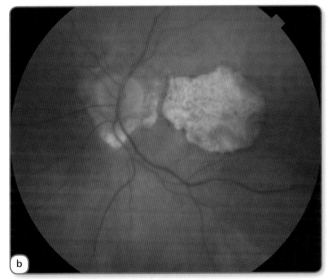

**Figure 12.2** Color fundus photographs (a) of the right eye and (b) of the left eye in a patient with extensive geographic atrophy from age-related macular degeneration. Note the central atrophy.

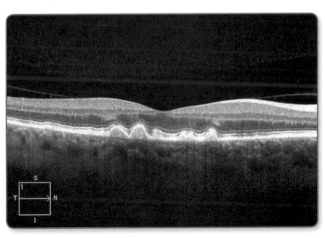

**Figure 12.3** Optical coherence tomography image of an eye with dry age-related macular degeneration. Note the presence of drusen between the retinal pigment epithelium and Bruch's membrane.

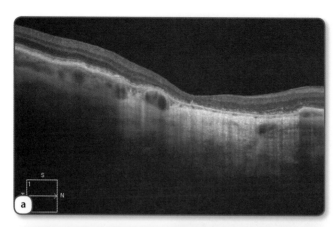

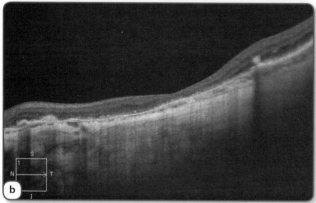

**Figure 12.4** Optical coherence tomography image (corresponding to color fundus photographs in Figure 12.2), (a) of the right eye and (b) of the left eye. Note the extensive outer retinal atrophy and absence of any intraretinal or subretinal fluid.

throughout the retina. Clinically drusen appear as yellow or white spots deep to the retina, specifically between Bruch's membrane and the RPE. Drusen are classified based on their size with small drusen being <63 μm, medium drusen between 63 and 125 μm, and large drusen being >125 μm. Hard drusen are small, common in normal eyes, and do not carry an increased risk for the development of neovascular ARMD. Soft drusen, however, are medium to large in size, may have nondiscrete borders or be confluent, and are associated with an increased risk of progression to neovascular ARMD or progressive atrophy.

Drusen themselves often do not cause decreased central vision; however, patients may have mildly impaired contrast sensitivity, metamorphopsia, and difficulty with light adaptation and reading.

Geographic atrophy is seen clinically as areas of hypopigmentation or depigmentation of the RPE and represents areas of outer retinal loss. Geographic atrophy often initially occurs in small (<1 DD) discrete areas but may coalesce over time. Visual acuity can be significantly affected if the damage extends through the fovea. Often these areas of geographic atrophy occur in a site of previous drusen.

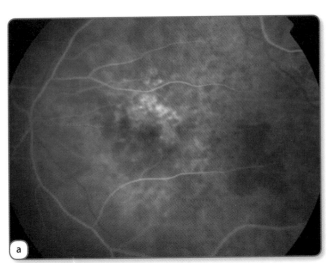

**Figure 12.5** (a–c) Fluorescein angiogram of an eye with dry macular degeneration. Note the extensive window defect, and absence of any choroidal neovascular membrane.

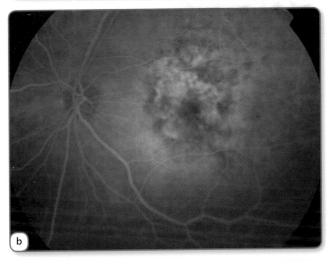

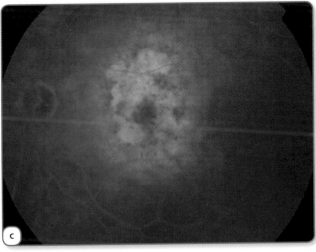

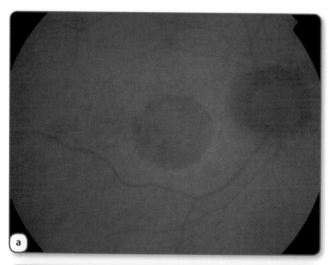

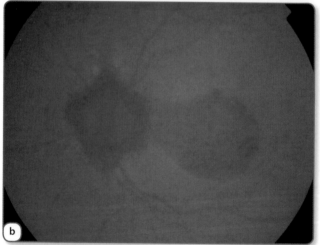

**Figure 12.6** Fundus autofluorescence (corresponding to color fundus photographs in Figure 12.2) (a) of the right eye and (b) of the left eye. Note the hypoautofluorescence in the area of geographic atrophy bilaterally.

## Treatment/prognosis/follow-up

There is no proven treatment for dry ARMD. Vitamin supplementation, dietary counseling, and cessation of smoking are the mainstays of treatment. The Age-Related Eye Disease Study (AREDS) and Age-Related Eye Disease Study 2 trial demonstrated that oral supplementation with vitamin C (500 mg), vitamin E (400 IU), zinc oxide (80 mg), cupric oxide (2 mg), lutein (10 mg), and zeaxanthin (2 mg) reduced the risk of progression to advanced dry ARMD and/or neovascular age-related macular degeneration by 25% over the course of 5 years in patients with moderate-to-severe dry ARMD.

The prognosis depends on the current appearance of the macula. There is a prognosis score that can be calculated. One point is given for each of the following: the presence of one large drusen or macular retinal pigment change for a maximum possible score of 4. The risk of progression to advanced ARMD depends on the initial risk score. With a score of 1 the 5-year risk is only 3%, a score of 2 is associated with a 12% risk, a score of 3 with a 25% risk, and with a score of 4, the risk increases to nearly 50%. Patients with dry macular degeneration should be followed every 3–12 months depending on the clinical status, and told to use an Amsler grid regularly at home. They should also be advised to report any changes in visual acuity immediately to their ophthalmologist, as this could signal a conversion to neovascular ARMD.

## Further reading

Age Related Eye Disease Research Group. Lutein + zeaxanthin and omega-3 fatty acids for age-related macular degeneration: the Age-Related Eye Disease Study 2 (AREDS) randomized clinical trial. JAMA 2013; 309:2005–15.

Ferris FL, Davis MD, Clemons TE, et al. A simplified severity scale for age-related macular degeneration: AREDS Report No. 18. Arch Ophthalmol 2005; 123:1570–74.

Yanoff M, Duker J. Ophthalmology, 3rd edn. London:Mosby Elsevier, 2009.

# 13

# Wet (exudative) age-related macular degeneration

## How to approach a patient with neovascularization within the macula associated with drusen or RPE changes

| Identify the primary pathologic clinical finding(s) | | |
|---|---|---|
| On fundoscopy there is the presence of subretinal pigment epithelial (RPE), subretinal and/or intraretinal fluid, retinal, subretinal or subRPE hemorrhage, lipid exudates, or a gray-green like membrane within the fovea in addition to macular drusen and RPE changes. | | |
| **Formulate a differential diagnosis** | | |
| **Most likely** | **Less likely** | **Least likely** |
| • Neovascular age-related macular degeneration (ARMD) | • Central serous chorioretinopathy, idiopathic choroidal neovascular membrane (CNV), Myopic CNV, CNV associated with angioid streaks, Bests disease | • Ocular histoplasmosis, North Carolina macular dystrophy, Doynes macular dystrophy, Sorsbys' macular dystrophy |
| **Query patient history** | | |
| • Is there a family history of ARMD or early onset vision loss?<br>• Any recent change in vision?<br>• Any previous history of intravitreal injections or laser treatment?<br>• What part of the country does the patient live currently and previously?<br>• Does the patient smoke cigarettes? | | |
| **Decide on ancillary diagnostic imaging** | | |
| Optical coherence tomography (OCT) is the main test utilized in the evaluation and treatment of neovascular ARMD. Additionally, fluorescein angiography is often used to confirm the initial diagnosis and evaluate the type of CNV present. | | |

## Ancillary diagnostic imaging interpretation

### Color fundus photography

Color fundus (CF) photography is not required for the treatment or management of neovascular ARMD. CF photography will demonstrate the presence of drusen, retinal pigmentary changes, intraretinal or subretinal hemorrhage, and CNV (**Figure 13.1**). Subretinal hyper-reflective material and dehiscences in the RPE are common.

### Optical coherence tomography

OCT is the main tool used to evaluate patients with neovascular ARMD. Intraretinal and subretinal fluid indicates the presence of active disease (**Figures 13.2** and **13.3**). OCT is also useful to monitor the clinical response over time.

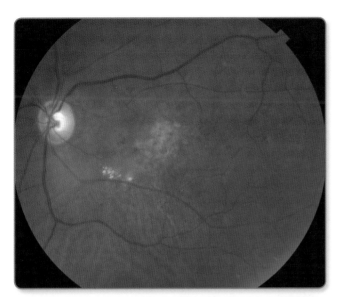

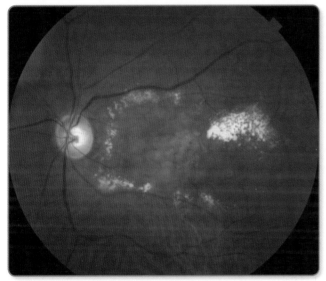

**Figure 15.1** Color fundus photographs of the left eye in a patient with idiopathic polypoidal choroidal vasculopathy. (a) Red polypoid lesions with soft exudates in the inferonasal macula and central atrophy. (b) Increasing exudate at 13 months.

## Fluorescein angiography

FA is not required to make the diagnosis of IPCV, as ICG angiography is typically more helpful. There will be pooling in the PEDs and areas of neurosensory detachment, and hyperfluorescence in the area of the choroidal vascular network may be evident. There may be blockage in areas of subretinal or sub-RPE hemorrhage, and window defects in areas of RPE atrophy.

## ICG angiography

ICG angiography is the most important diagnostic test in this condition. There is early hyperfluorescence of the choroidal vascular network

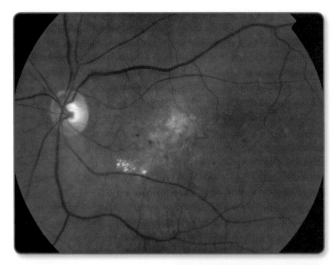

**Figure 15.2** Red-free photograph of the left eye from the same patient as in Figure 15.1 that highlights the exudates and hemorrhages that can be more difficult to appreciate in the color photos and clinically.

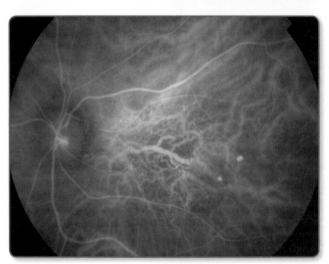

**Figure 15.3** Indocyanine green angiography from the same patient as in Figure 15.1 demonstrating late hyperfluorescence of the polypoidal lesions in the temporal and nasal macula, which correspond to the reddish polypoid lesions in Figure 15.1.

with later hyperfluorescence of the polyps at the edges of the network, which may leak (**Figure 15.3**). Notably, there is absence of a staining plaque in the late phases that is characteristic of an occult CNV. It may also be useful in guiding photodynamic therapy.

## Final diagnosis: idiopathic polypoidal choroidal vasculopathy

### Epidemiology/etiology

IPCV, initially named 'posterior uveal bleeding syndrome,' was first described in African American women. It is more common in pigmented races and females. It typically presents between 50 and 65 years of age. Alternatively, it can be a variant of wet AMD. The critical finding is a dilated network of inner choroidal vessels that intermittently leak, leading to serosanguineous neurosensory and RPE detachments. The pathogenesis is not completely understood, although hypertension has been implicated in possibly contributing to choroidal vascular dilatation.

## Symptoms and clinical findings

Patients may present with blurred vision, scotomas, or metamorphopsia. If the central macula is spared, the patient may be asymptomatic. Eventually, both eyes are usually affected, though unilateral disease has been reported. Serosanguineous neurosensory and pigment epithelial detachments are the classic findings. Red-orange subretinal lesions may be evident, particularly if there is overlying RPE atrophy. These lesions are classically in the peripapillary or macular area; however, unlike in AMD, extramacular involvement may occur. The absence of drusen or disciform scars helps distinguish this disease from AMD. Vitreous hemorrhage and secondary CNV have been reported but are uncommon.

## Treatment/prognosis/follow-up

Patients with IPCV can present as either a variant of wet AMD or as a primary disorder. Distinguishing between IPCV and typical CNV associated with AMD is important as each carries a different prognosis and responds differently to treatment. Many cases of IPCV without macular involvement can be observed. For those with symptomatic macular involvement, treatment options include anti-VEGF therapy and/or photodynamic therapy. Patients with IPCV seem to have a less robust response to anti-VEGF agents as compared to patients with AMD. The EVEREST trial demonstrated that patients with the IPCV variant of wet AMD treated with combined therapy with monthly ranibizumab and photodynamic therapy had higher rates of polyp regression than either therapy alone. At 6 months, the combination therapy group showed a trend toward more letters gained than either monotherapy group; however, this study was not powered to detect visual acuity differences.

Roughly half of untreated patients have a relatively good visual prognosis with visual acuity of better than 20/30. The other half of patients end up with vision worse than 20/100. Visual acuity at the time of presentation is the best predictor of final acuity. End-stage disciform scars are uncommon in IPCV.

# Further reading

Koh A, Lee WK, Chen LJ, et al. EVEREST Study: efficacy and safety of verteporfin photodynamic therapy in combination with ranibizumab or alone versus ranibizumab monotherapy in patients with symptomatic macular polypoidal choroidal vasculopathy. Retina 2012; 32:1453-64.

Spaide RD, Donsoff I, Lam DL, et al. Treatment of polypoidal choroidal vasculopathy with photodynamic therapy. Retina 2002; 22:529–35.

Spaide RD, Yannuzzi LA, Slakter JS, et al. Indocyanine green videoangiography of idiopathic polypoidal choroidal vasculopathy. Retina 1995; 15:100–110.

Uyama M, Wada M, Nagai Y, et al. Polypoidal choroidal vasculopathy: natural history. Am J Ophthalmol 2002; 133:639–48.

Yannuzzi LA, Ciardella A, Spaide RF, et al. The expanding clinical spectrum of idiopathic polypoidal choroidal vasculopathy. Arch Ophthalmol 1997; 115:478–85.

Yannuzzi LA, Sorenson J, Spaide RF, Lipson B. Idiopathic polypoidal choroidal vasculopathy (IPCV). Retina 1990; 10:1–8.

# Retinal angiomatous proliferation

## How to approach a patient with telangiectatic vessels, exudate, and a retinal pigment epithelial detachment

| Identify the primary pathologic clinical finding(s) | | |
|---|---|---|
| There is prominent retinal vasculature, intraretinal hemorrhage, hard exudate, and a pigment epithelial detachment. | | |
| Formulate a differential diagnosis | | |
| **Most likely** | **Less likely** | **Least likely** |
| • Retinal angiomatous proliferation (RAP) | • Neovascular age-related macular degeneration (ARMD), idiopathic polypoidal choroidal vasculopathy (IPCV), choroidal neovascularization (CNV) | • Macular telangiectasia type II, adult onset vitelliform dystrophy |
| Query patient history | | |
| • Is there a family history of ARMD or early onset vision loss?<br>• Any recent change in vision?<br>• Any previous history of intravitreal injections or treatment for ARMD?<br>• Does the patient smoke cigarettes? | | |
| Decide on ancillary diagnostic imaging | | |
| ARMD is diagnosed based on clinical examination but can be followed over time with fundus photography and optical coherence tomography (OCT). Classification of the various subtypes of neovascular ARMD, specifically RAP, however, requires a combination of OCT, fluorescein angiography, and indocyanine green (ICG) angiography for accurate diagnosis and evaluation of response to treatment. | | |

## Ancillary diagnostic imaging interpretation

### Color fundus photography

Color fundus photography is not required for diagnosis but can be used for clinical documentation as well as to assess the disease over time. RAP lesions typically demonstrate intraretinal hemorrhages, hard exudates, and a pigment epithelial detachment (**Figure 16.1**).

### Optical coherence tomography

OCT in a RAP lesion typically demonstrates fluid in all three spaces: sub-RPE (RPED), subretinal, and intraretinal. In most cases, the intraretinal fluid predominates (**Figure 16.2**). OCT, as with classic ARMD, is used for baseline evaluation as well as to monitor response to therapy.

### Fluorescein angiography

Fluorescein angiography imaging in early stages may be helpful to detect intraretinal neovascularization, and in late stages can reveal occult or minimally classic leakage (**Figure 16.3**).

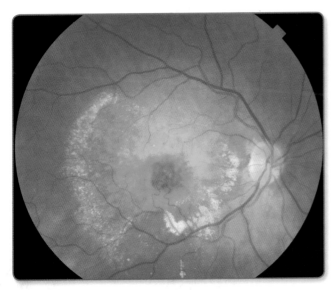

**Figure 16.1** Color fundus photograph of the right eye in a patient with a retinal angiomatous proliferation lesion. Note the central elevated PED with retinal-choroidal anastomosis at the inferior edge. There is associated retinal thickening, small areas of intraretinal hemorrhage, and surrounding exudate in a circinate pattern.

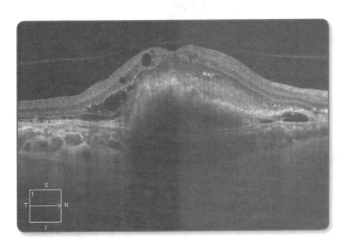

**Figure 16.2** Optical coherence tomographic images from the same patient as in Figure 16.1. Note the fibrovascular PED with overlying intraretinal cystic changes and hyper-reflective subretinal material. Note also the presence of a thick choroid that is not found in typical age-related macular degeneration.

## ICG angiography

ICG angiography is the most important diagnostic test in evaluation of patients with a RAP lesion, and the lesions or polys show up as focal 'hot spots' of hyperfluorescence (**Figure 16.4**). Specifically, high-speed ICG angiography can localize the retinal feeding arterioles and draining venules.

## Final diagnosis: RAP

### Epidemiology/etiology

RAP (type III CNV) is considered a distinct form of neovascular ARMD in which new vessels originate from within the retina and create a

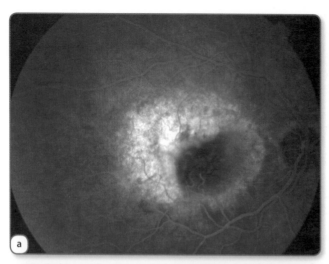

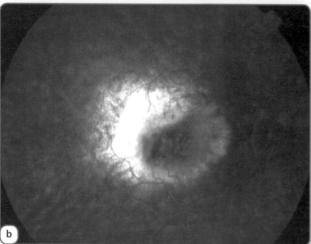

**Figure 16.3** Early (a) and late (b) fluorescein angiography images in a patient with a retinal angiomatous proliferation lesion. Note the late leakage temporal to the fovea in addition to proliferation of retinal vessels within the fovea.

surrounding telangiectatic response, potentially communicating with a deeper CNV, instead of arising from the choroidal circulation. Initially described as a 'retinal angiomatous lesion' in 1992 by Hartnett, it was further characterized by Yannuzzi in 2001 as a type 3 neovascularization. In contrast to an occult (type 1) or classic (type 2) CNV, RAP is an intraretinal neovascularization that tends to develop bilaterally in the paramacular area. It is more common in Caucasian females, and compared to the common form of neovascular ARMD, is more often found in older individuals over 80 years of age.

## Symptoms and clinical findings

Vision loss in RAP is due to aberrant blood vessel growth within or beneath the retina. Clinical manifestations include preretinal and intraretinal hemorrhage, exudates, intraretinal edema, and PED

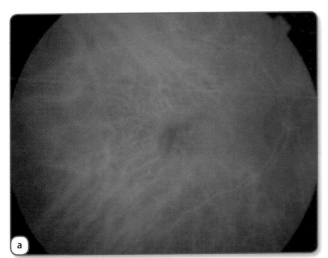

**Figure 16.4** Indocyanine green angiographic images highlight the multifocal areas of hyperfluorescence over the PED in early (a) and late (b) images.

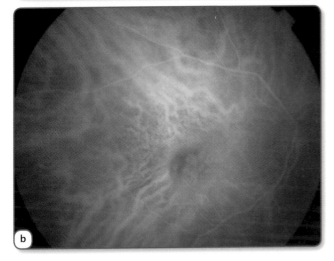

formation. As such, symptoms of RAP lesions may be similar to those with other types of neovascular ARMD and are related to the location and extent of vascular leakage.

RAP is further subclassified into three stages, including intraretinal neovascularization (stage 1), subretinal vascularization (stage 2), and retinal-choroidal anastomosis with CNV (stage 3). Identification of intraretinal neovascularization can be difficult, and as such, most cases are stage 3 at the time of diagnosis.

## Treatment/prognosis/follow-up

There has been some debate as to whether RAP has a less favorable outcome compared to the more common types of neovascular ARMD. There are no randomized clinical trials for treatment of RAP lesions, but therapies have been tried with variable success, including laser photocoagulation, transpupillary thermotherapy, and surgical removal. Conventional laser photocoagulation may work for treating early stage RAP outside the fovea. Once the lesion progresses, however, it is more difficult to treat. PDT with and without intravitreal steroids has been used with some success. Finally, anti-VEGF agents have shown promise with decreased macular edema and improved visual function.

## Further reading

Gupta B, Jyothi S, Sivaprasad S. Current treatment options for retinal angiomatous proliferans (RAP). Br J Ophthalmol 2010; 94:672–7.

Polito A, Napolitano MC, Bandelo F, Chiodini RR. The role of optical coherence tomography (OCT) in the diagnosis and management of retinal angiomatous proliferation (RAP) in patients with age-related macular degeneration. Ann Acad Med Singapore 2006; 35:420–24.

Yannuzzi LA, Negrao S, Lida T, et al. Retinal angiomatous proliferate in age-related macular degeneration. Retina 2001; 21:416–24.

# How to approach a patient with reticular and/or vitelliform-like retinal pigment epithelial changes without drusen

| Identify the primary pathologic clinical finding(s) | | |
|---|---|---|
| There are reticular pigment changes within the macula with the notable absence of drusen. The changes may take on different shapes. There may be yellow subretinal vitelliform lesions that appear hyper fluorescent on autofluorescence. | | |
| **Formulate a differential diagnosis** | | |
| **Most likely** | **Less likely** | **Least likely** |
| • Pattern dystrophy of the retinal pigment epithelium | • Adult-onset vitelliform macular dystrophy, dry age-related macular degeneration, Stargardt's disease, Best disease | • Cuticular drusen, pseudovitelliform dystrophies, maternally inherited diabetes, and deafness |
| **Query patient history** | | |
| • Any family history of vision loss early in life?<br>• Any history of previous injections or lasers?<br>• Any recent decrease in vision? | | |
| **Decide on ancillary diagnostic imaging** | | |
| Pattern dystrophy is a clinical diagnosis that is confirmed by ancillary testing and, occasionally, genetic testing. Color fundus (CF) photographs may be used for documentation purposes but are not required for diagnosis. Optical coherence tomography (OCT) is helpful to rule out intra or subretinal fluid. Fundus autofluorescence (FAF) and fluorescein angiography (FA) may be helpful in ambiguous cases. | | |

# Ancillary diagnostic imaging interpretation

## CF photography

CF photography demonstrates areas of retinal pigment epithelium (RPE) hyperpigmentation and RPE changes. There is notable absence of drusen or yellow flecks (**Figure 17.1**). A yellow vitelliform lesion may be present.

## Optical coherence tomography

OCT has a very characteristic pattern in pattern dystrophy. There is typically hyporeflectivity between the IS/OS (inner segment/outer segment) junction and the RPE, which is not associated with subretinal fluid or active leakage (**Figure 17.2**). There may also be focal disruptions in the IS/OS junction and areas of hyper-reflectivity in the border between Bruch's membrane and RPE.

## Fluorescein angiography

FA will demonstrate blockage from areas of retina pigment epithelial clumping without evidence of choroidal neovascular membrane (**Figure 17.3**).

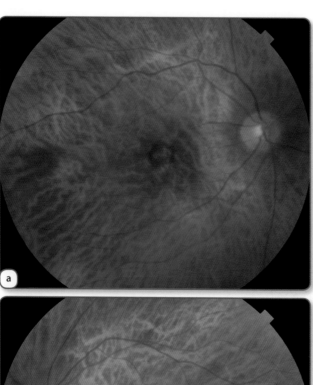

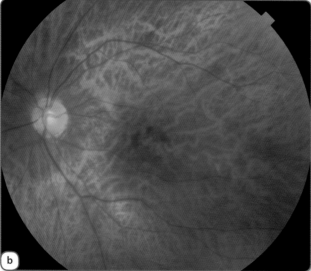

**Figure 17.1** Color fundus photographs of the right (a) and left eyes (b) in a patient with pattern dystrophy. Note the retinal pigment epithelium pigment clumping and notable absence of drusen.

## Indocyanine green angiography

Indocyanine green angiography (ICGA) can be helpful to evaluate for choroidal neovascularization or polypoidal lesion that might be missed on FA (**Figure 17.4**). ICGA is not necessary for the diagnosis but is helpful to rule out other causes such as idiopathic polypoidal choroidal vasculopathy and central serous chorioretinopathy.

## Fundus autofluorescence

FAF will demonstrate mixed areas of hyperautofluorescence (accumulation of lipofuscin) and areas of hypoautofluorescence (**Figure 17.5**).

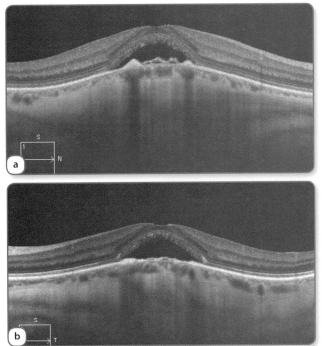

**Figure 17.2** Enhanced depth optical coherence tomography images of right (a) and left eyes (b) in a patient with pattern dystrophy. Note the focal area of hyporeflectivity between IS/OS (inner segment/outer segment) junction and the retinal pigment epithelium (RPE) that does not represent subretinal fluid. There is also hyper-reflective material that appears as focal excrescences originating from the RPE toward the IS/OS junction in (a). Also note some focal disruption of the IS/OS junction in both eyes.

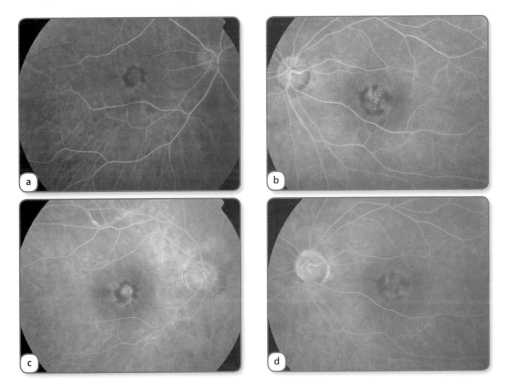

**Figure 17.3** Fluorescein angiogram of the right (a, c) and left eyes (b, d) in a patient with pattern dystrophy. (a) and (b) are early images and (c) and (d) are late images. Note the areas of hypofluorescence in the early images corresponding to retinal pigment epithelium hyperpigmentation and some late staining in the right eye more than the left. Note the absence of any late leakage, which would be consistent with choroidal neovascularization.

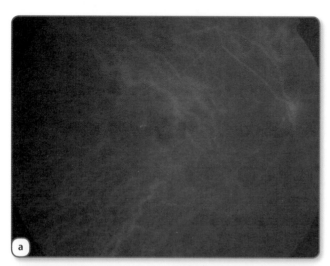

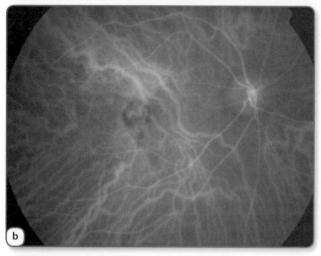

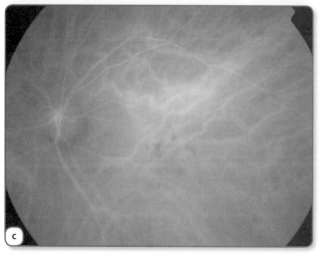

**Figure 17.4** Indocyanine green angiography of the right (a, b) and left eyes (c) in a patient with pattern dystrophy. (a) Represents early images; (b) and (c) are late images. Note the absence of any choroidal neovascular membrane or polypoidal choroidal lesions. There is some blockage from retinal pigment epithelium clumping more notable in the right eye than the left.

# Final diagnosis: pattern dystrophy

## Epidemiology/etiology

Pattern dystrophy refers to a group of disorders that share a common genetic defect. The mutation occurs in the RDS gene (peripherin 2, PRPHS), which encodes a trans-membrane glycoprotein that is found in the photoreceptor outer segment disks and is thought to play a role in the photoreceptor's structural integrity. This group of disorders is autosomal dominant with incomplete penetrance and variable expressivity. Depending on the specific gene defect, there are various phenotypes that may look quite different clinically. Clinically distinct manifestations of pattern dystrophy include reticular dystrophy of the RPE, butterfly-shaped dystrophy, adult onset vitelliform macular dystrophy (synonyms include adult onset foveomacular dystrophy,

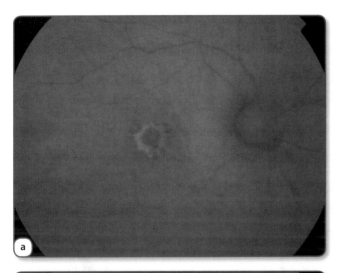

**Figure 17.5** Fundus autofluorescence of the right (a) and left eyes (b) in a patient with pattern dystrophy. Note the classic appearance with mixed areas of hyperautofluorescence and hypoautofluorescence.

adult Best disease, adult onset foveal pigment epithelial dystrophy), and a dystrophy simulating Stargardt's disease.

Subretinal deposits that exhibit fundus hyperautofluorescence appear typically in the third to fifth decades of life. On FA there is early blockage and late staining of the lesion.

The differential diagnosis of pattern dystrophies also includes Best disease and pseudovitelliform dystrophies. Best disease is an autosomal dominant disorder with variable penetrance and expressivity. There is accumulation of lipofuscin in the retinal pigment epithelium and/or subretinal space secondary to a mutation in the VMD 2 gene, which encodes the protein bestrophin. This is typically a childhood disease and an abnormal EOG is diagnostic. Pseudovitelliform lesions look clinically similar to Best disease with the presence of yellow subretinal material; however, there is no associated bestrophin mutation.

## Symptoms and clinical findings

Most patients with pattern dystrophy are asymptomatic and are discovered incidentally upon routine ophthalmic examination. Affected individuals may complain of decreased vision or metamorphopsia. Many are referred to retina specialists for evaluation of macular degeneration. Clinical findings include hyperpigmentation and retinal pigment epithelial clumping in the macula without associated yellow flecks or drusen.

## Treatment/prognosis/follow-up

Visual acuity is usually good for the first five to six decades of life, and the prognosis for maintaining good visual acuity is excellent, with the exception of patients that develop geographic atrophy later in life. There is a small risk of choroidal neovascularization; however, this is lower than in age-related macular degeneration. The CNV associated with pattern dystrophy appears to be less aggressive than those associated with wet AMD.

# Further reading

Franchis PJ, Schultz DW, Gregory AM, et al. Genetic and phenotypic heterogeneity in pattern dystrophy. Br J Ophthalmol 2005; 89:1115–9.

Hsieh RC, Fine BS, Lyons JS. Pattern dystrophies of the retinal pigment epithelium. Arch Ophthalmol 1977; 95:429–35.

Marmor MF, Byers B. Pattern dystrophy of the pigment epithelium. Am J Ophthalmol 1977; 84:32–44.

## How to approach a patient with irregular striations radiating from the optic nerve

| Identify the primary pathologic clinical finding(s) | | |
|---|---|---|
| There are irregular lines radiating from the optic nerve head that are variable in size and shape and may range from 50 to 500 μm. There may be evidence of macular atrophy, and reticular RPE changes particularly if a choroidal neovascular membrane has previously been present. | | |
| **Formulate a differential diagnosis** | | |
| **Most likely** | **Less likely** | **Least likely** |
| • Angioid streaks, lacquer cracks secondary to pathologic myopia | • Choroidal rupture, choroidal folds, central serous chorioretinopathy | • Toxoplasmosis, histoplasmosis, choroidal tumor |
| **Query patient history** | | |
| • Does the patient have a history of ocular trauma?<br>• Has the patient previously had intraocular surgery?<br>• Is the patient near sighted?<br>• Any history of previous vision loss?<br>• Does the patient have any systemic medical conditions?<br>• Does the patient have a rash on their neck? | | |
| **Decide on ancillary diagnostic imaging** | | |
| The diagnosis of angioid streaks is made clinically based on characteristic findings on dilated fundus examination. Fluorescein angiography (FA) can be used to confirm the diagnosis in ambiguous cases as well as evaluate for choroidal neovascular membrane. | | |

## Ancillary diagnostic imaging interpretation

### Color photography

Angioid streaks appear as bilateral irregular lines, deep to the retina, which are brownish orange (and sometimes very subtle) and radiate from the optic nerve (**Figure 18.1**). Peripapillary atrophy may be present.

### Optical coherence tomography

Optical coherence tomography (OCT) can be used to evaluate for the presence of CNV which presents with subretinal and/or intraretinal fluid (**Figure 18.2**). OCT can also be used to monitor response to therapy in conjunction with FA.

### Fluorescein angiography

FA is very helpful in the diagnosis of angioid streaks, particularly when clinically subtle. FA will demonstrate late staining of the linear striations radiating from the optic nerve, and evaluate for the presence of active CNV (**Figure 18.3**).

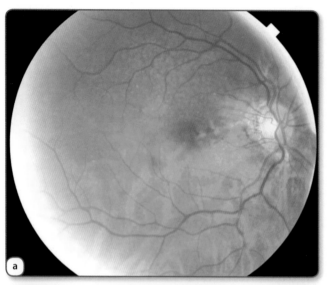

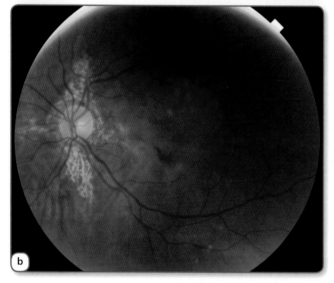

**Figure 18.1** Color fundus photographs in a patient with angioid streaks in the (a) right eye and (b) left eye. In the left eye note the presence of retinal hemorrhage and blunted foveal reflex suggestive of active CNV. Note the presence of linear striations off of the optic nerve in both eyes and macular RPE changes. CNV, choroidal neovascular membrane.

# Final diagnosis: angioid streaks

## Epidemiology/etiology

The pathophysiology of angioid streaks is not well understood. Angioid streaks occur from breaks in Bruch's membrane and histopathologic studies have demonstrated the presence of calcification and thickening in Bruch's membrane and adjacent interstitial space with fragmentation of the elastic fibers. Ingrowth of fibrovascular tissue can occur into the subretinal space through these areas of weakness leading to retinal hemorrhage and choroidal neovascularization.

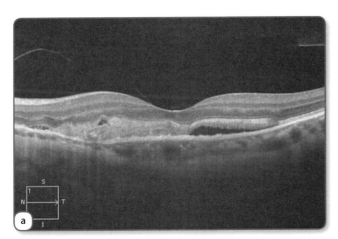

**Figure 18.2** Optical coherence tomographic imaging of a CNV associated with angioid streaks (corresponding to Figure 18.1b). Part (a) is the five-line raster scan and (b) is the macular cube scan. Note the presence of subretinal fluid as well as choroidal neovascularization under the retina.

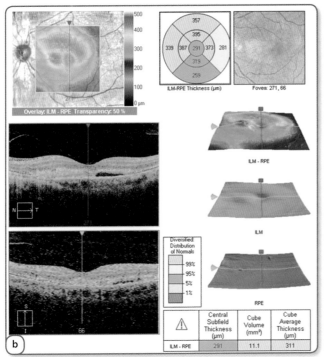

There is no gender or racial predilections for angioid streaks; however, there are a number of systemic associations including Pseudoxanthoma elasticum, Ehlers–Danlos syndrome, Paget's disease, sickle cell disease, and other hemoglobinopathies. Systemic disease is found in about 50% of people who present with angioid streaks. Less common associations include abetalipoproteinemia, acromegaly, diabetes mellitus, facial angiomatosis, hemochromatosis, hemolytic anemia, hereditary spherocytosis, hypercalcinosis, hyperphosphatemia, lead poisoning, myopia, neurofibromatosis, senile elastosis, Sturge–Weber syndrome,

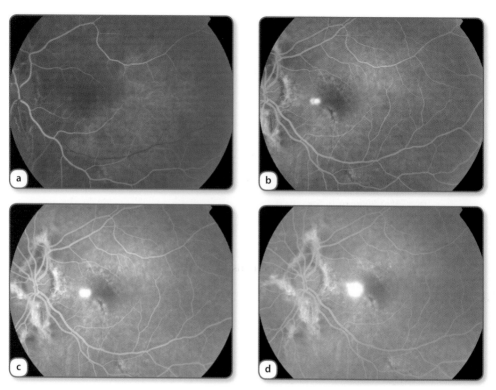

**Figure 18.3** (a–d) Fluorescein angiogram of the left eye (corresponding to Figure 18.1b). Note the presence of active CNV that is seen as early staining with late leakage nasal to the fovea. Note also the presence of staining of the angioid streaks radiating off the optic nerve.

and tuberous sclerosis. Angioid streaks are also associated with optic nerve head drusen. Because of this, patients without a known systemic disease should be worked up by their primary care doctor and receive a complete physical examination, skin biopsy, and blood tests to evaluate levels of serum alkaline phosphatase, serum calcium and phosphate, and hemoglobin electrophoresis.

## Symptoms and clinical findings

Patients with angioid streaks are asymptomatic unless they develop associated choroidal neovascularization, in which case they may present with decreased vision and metamorphopsia. The majority of patients with angioid streaks will ultimately develop CNV and bilateral disease is the rule. Clinical findings of angioid streaks include linear radiations extending from the optic nerve head that may be associated with peripapillary atrophy. If there is active CNV or a previous history of CNV then there are likely macular RPE changes as well. There may also be the classic finding of 'peau d'orange' in which the retina appears similar to the skin of an orange.

## Treatment/prognosis/follow-up

There is no proven treatment to reduce the risk of development of CNV in patients with angioid streaks except to avoid ocular trauma. Patients are sometimes advised to avoid contact sports and to wear safety glasses.

Treatment is performed when there is CNV that occurs in conjunction with angioid streaks. Options for treatment include focal laser, photodynamic therapy, and intravitreal injections with anti-VEGF agents such as bevacizumab and ranibizumab. Focal laser is utilized less often in the age of anti-VEGF therapy, as there is about 77% risk of recurrence and poor long-term visual results. Most retina specialists use focal laser only for small, localized extrafoveal CNV. Similarly, the data on PDT therapy in CNV related to angioid streaks suggest poor results, and therefore PDT is not considered first-line therapy but may be considered for combination therapy with anti-VEGF agents. Intravitreal anti-VEGF therapy is considered the treatment of choice. In a number of small case series, the majority (87–100%) of bevacizumab-treated patients demonstrated visual stabilization or improvement. Similar excellent visual results were observed in patients treated with ranibizumab. Unlike AMD, with angioid streaks there may be acute worsening from the injection itself. Case reports have been published illustrating expansion of the angioid streaks after anti-VEGF therapy. There also may be persistent subretinal fluid on OCT with inactivity on FA, making treatment decisions challenging. Regardless of treatment modality, CNV recurrence is common and occurred in about 33% of eyes at 19-month follow-up.

## Further reading

Clarkson JG, Altman RD. Angioid streaks. Surv Ophthalmol 1982; 26:235–46.
Ryan S, Sadda S, Hinton D, et al. Retina, 5th edn. Philadelphia, PA: Elsevier, 2013:1267–73.
Yanoff M, Duker JS. Ophthalmology, 4th edn. Philadelphia, PA: Elsevier, 2014:600–604.
Yanuzzi LA. The Retinal Atlas. Philadelphia, PA: Elsevier, 2010:516–18.

# How to approach a patient with posterior staphyloma and macular degeneration

| Identify the primary pathologic clinical finding(s) | | |
|---|---|---|
| There is progressive axial elongation with posterior staphyloma formation and secondary macular degeneration. | | |
| **Formulate a differential diagnosis** | | |
| **Most likely** | **Less likely** | **Least likely** |
| • Myopic degeneration | • Age-related macular degeneration | • Ocular histoplasmosis |
| **Query patient history** | | |
| • Is the patient near sighted?<br>• Is there any history of macular degeneration in the family?<br>• Has the patient ever had a laser or injection? | | |
| **Decide on ancillary diagnostic imaging** | | |
| The diagnosis is made based on characteristic posterior segment findings in a myopic individual. | | |

# Ancillary diagnostic imaging interpretation

## Color photography

Color photography is not required for diagnosis, but can be used to demonstrate areas of RPE atrophy, which may be focal or diffuse, as well as the presence of posterior staphyloma (**Figure 19.1**).

## Optical coherence tomography

Optical coherence tomography (OCT) is helpful for evaluation of CNV or associated myopic macular schisis. CNV may demonstrate an elevated lesion in the subretinal space; however, there is often an absence of subretinal or intraretinal fluid in myopic CNV, which is different than typical CNV associated with macular degeneration (**Figure 19.2**).

## Fluorescein angiography

Fluorescein angiography may demonstrate a focal area of increasing hyperfluorescence (**Figure 19.3**). For small CNV in particular, FA can be a powerful tool for detection.

## Indocyanine green angiography

Indocyanine green angiography (ICGA) may not be helpful in delineating a myopic CNV. Typical CNV will be hyperfluorescent on ICGA; however, this is not necessarily true of myopic CNV.

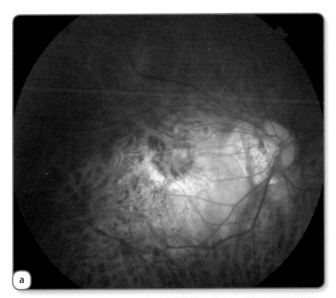

**Figure 19.1** Color fundus photograph of a patient with myopic degeneration of the right (a) and left eyes (b). Note the tilted optic nerve with peripapillary atrophy. Notice the diffuse chorioretinal atrophy and RPE changes in the right eye with areas that are concerning for possible choroidal neovascular membrane.

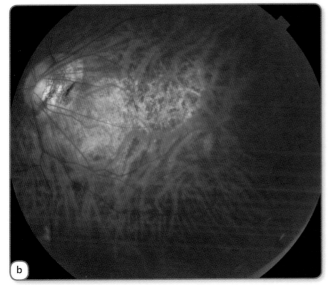

# Final diagnosis: myopic degeneration

## Epidemiology/etiology

Myopic degeneration occurs in eyes with >6 D of myopia; however, not all eyes with pathologic myopia undergo myopic degeneration. The prevalence in the United States is 2.1%, with women affected twice as often as men. There is a higher incidence of myopia among Asian individuals, particularly from East Asia. The pathophysiology of this progressive and degenerative disorder is largely unknown, there may

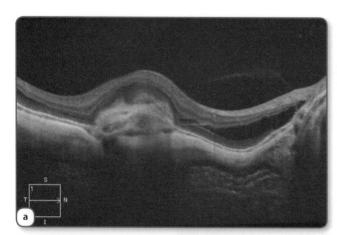

**Figure 19.2** Optical coherence tomography through the macula in a patient with myopic degeneration of the right (a) and left eyes (b). In the right eye, note the presence of subretinal elevation consistent with myopic CNV. There is also myopic schisis nasally in the right eye. In the left eye, there is no evidence of myopic CNV.

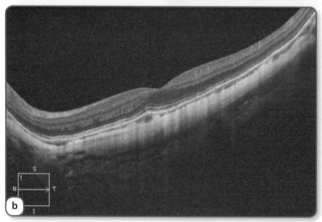

be some degree of scleral growth and remodeling that occurs, and there are likely genetic and environmental factors. Pathologic myopia and myopic degeneration are associated with systemic syndromes such as Stickler's, Ehlers–Danlos, and Marfan's. Myopic degeneration causes vision loss earlier in life than typical age-related macular degeneration.

## Symptoms and clinical findings

Patients may be asymptomatic until they present with acute metamorphopsia and photopsias when a break in Bruch's membrane or a CNV occurs.

Patients with myopic degeneration or pathologic myopia are at increased risk of cataract formation, open angle glaucoma, rhegmatogenous retinal detachment, and vitreous detachment at a younger age.

Posterior staphyloma, which is the classic ocular finding in myopic degeneration, is an ectasia of the sclera, and occurs more commonly superotemporally. Stretching of the sclera causes progressive thinning of the overlying retina, RPE, and choroid. Bruch's membrane is

# 20

# Full-thickness macular hole

## How to approach a patient with an apparent full-thickness foveal defect

| Identify the primary pathologic clinical finding(s) | | |
|---|---|---|
| On examination, the patient has what appears to be a full-thickness retinal defect in the center of the macula (**Figure 20.1**). | | |
| Formulate a differential diagnosis | | |
| **Most likely** | **Less likely** | **Least likely** |
| • Full-thickness macular hole (FTMH), lamellar macular hole, cystoid macular edema, pseudohole associated with epiretinal membrane | • Vitreomacular traction syndrome | • Localized macular scar |
| Query patient history | | |
| • Has there been recent blunt trauma?<br>• Is the patient experiencing any metamorphopsia?<br>• When was the visual problem first noted and has it been gradual or sudden in onset?<br>• How severe is the visual impairment – is it affecting the patient's ability to perform any activities? | | |
| Decide on ancillary diagnostic imaging | | |
| Optical coherence tomography (OCT) is the best diagnostic test to confirm the presence of a macular hole. Fluorescein angiography, though historically useful, now has limited utility in macular hole evaluation, as it is unnecessarily invasive and provides less insight than OCT. | | |

## Ancillary diagnostic imaging interpretation

### Optical coherence tomography

OCT shows a full-thickness macular defect involving the fovea with a visible overlying operculum and localized separation of the posterior hyaloid (**Figures 20.2** and **20.3**). OCT has become the gold standard for confirming the diagnosis of a FTMH. OCT is also helpful in monitoring progress following surgical intervention.

## Final diagnosis: full-thickness idiopathic macular hole, stage 4

### Epidemiology/etiology

Middle-aged females between 50 and 70 years of age are most commonly affected. Macular holes develop as a result of progressive pathological perifoveal vitreous separation with adherence to the fovea. There is a spectrum of disease progression including premacular hole (stage 0 or vitreomacular adhesion), impending macular hole (stages 1A and 1B or vitreomacular traction) and FTMH (stages 2–4). FTMHs can be further categorized as small, medium, and large based on aperture size

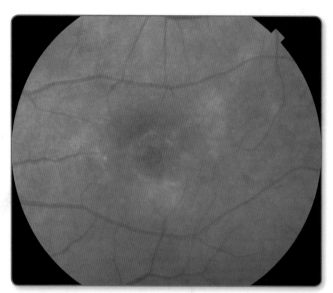

**Figure 20.1** Color fundus photograph of a full-thickness macular hole. There is a central, circular retinal defect and shallow surrounding cuff of subretinal fluid.

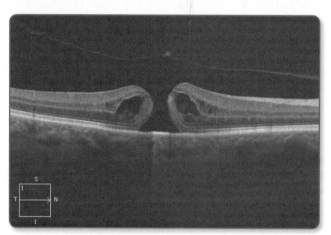

**Figure 20.2** Optical coherence tomography of a small stage 4 full-thickness macular hole. There is a full-thickness defect of the central macula and intraretinal cystic spaces on the edges of the hole. There is a free-floating operculum in the vitreous cavity that is attached to the posterior hyaloid.

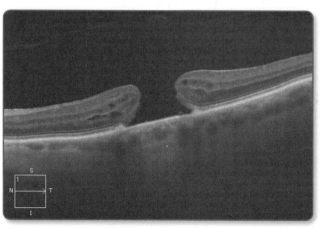

**Figure 20.3** Optical coherence tomography of a large stage 4 full-thickness macular hole.

as measured with OCT. Stage 2 and 3 FTMHs have concurrent VMT, while stage 4 FTMHs do not have VMT. Pre- and impending macular holes spontaneously resolve in a large percentage of eyes. FTMHs are important to distinguish clinically because these are highly unlikely to resolve spontaneously, and intervention should be considered.

## Symptoms and clinical findings

Patients typically present with decreased central visual acuity in the involved eye, ranging from mild (20/40) to severe (Count Fingers). A FTMH is characterized by a circular defect of the retina in the central fovea exposing the underlying bare retinal pigment epithelium. The size of the defect can range from small to larger than 500 μm. Patients may note a central gap of light when a slit beam is positioned directly over the hole (positive Watzke-Allen sign). The absence of concurrent vitreomacular traction on OCT is important to note, as this influences treatment options.

## Treatment/prognosis/follow-up

Intravitreal ocriplasmin or surgical intervention with pars plana vitrectomy may be considered in small or medium FTMHs with concurrent VMT. In larger holes and holes without VMT, surgical intervention is recommended. A standard surgical approach includes pars plana vitrectomy with creation of a complete posterior vitreous detachment, often with peeling of the internal limiting membrane around the edge of the hole, and gas tamponade with sulfur hexafluoride (SF6) or perfluoropropane (C3F8). Postoperative face down positioning is sometimes advocated for up to 7 days depending on the diameter of the hole and surgeon preference. Success of primary surgical intervention decreases with chronicity and size of macular hole. Late reopening of surgically repaired macular holes can occur even years after successful closure and it is thought that peeling of the internal limiting membrane at the time of primary repair decreases this risk.

# 21

# Lamellar macular hole

## How to approach a patient with a round, reddish lesion in the fovea

| Identify the primary pathologic clinical finding(s) | | |
|---|---|---|
| There is a well-demarcated, round, reddish irregularity in the fovea that appears to be partial thickness. | | |
| **Formulate a differential diagnosis** | | |
| Most likely | Less likely | Least likely |
| • Lamellar macular hole and macular pseudohole | • Full-thickness macular hole | • Cystoid macular edema, pattern dystrophy, acute macular neuroretinopathy, Valsalva retinopathy |
| **Query patient history** | | |
| • Is there any impairment in visual acuity?<br>• Is metamorphopsia present?<br>• Has there been recent trauma or surgery on the eye? | | |
| **Decide on ancillary diagnostic imaging** | | |
| Optical coherence tomography (OCT) is the most useful imaging modality to detect abnormalities of the fovea and can easily reveal the extent of involvement of various layers of the retina. | | |

## Ancillary diagnostic imaging interpretation

### Optical coherence tomography

OCT shows disruption of the normal foveal depression with a partial thickness retinal defect involving the fovea (**Figures 21.1** and **21.2**). Schisis or intraretinal layer splitting is present, often symmetrically on each edge of the fovea. The schisis typically occurs between the outer plexiform and outer nuclear layers. The photoreceptor layer is conspicuously present, which helps to distinguish this entity from full-thickness macular hole.

## Final diagnosis: lamellar macular hole

### Epidemiology/etiology

Lamellar macular holes may represent an abortive step toward full-thickness macular hole formation due to vitreomacular tractional forces, although other pathophysiologic mechanisms have also been implicated such as epiretinal membrane contraction or ruptured cysts in the setting of cystoid macular edema. Prior to the advent of OCT, clinical examination findings and historical features were the basis for diagnosis, which was unreliable. OCT now allows for standardization in diagnosis by identifying four basic features common in lamellar macular holes: (1) irregular foveal configuration, (2) an inner foveal breach, (3) schisis between the outer plexiform and nuclear layers, and (4) an intact underlying photoreceptor layer. The concurrent presence of epiretinal membrane (ERM) is commonly seen with lamellar macular holes.

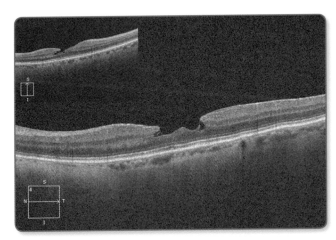

**Figure 21.1** Optical coherence tomography (OCT) of lamellar macular hole. OCT shows typical features of lamellar macular hole including an irregular foveal contour with loss of inner retinal tissue, schisis (inset), and an intact underlying photoreceptor layer. There is a mild concurrent epiretinal membrane.

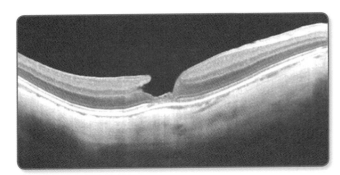

**Figure 21.2** Optical coherence tomography of lamellar macular hole. Another example of a typical lamellar hole with an irregular fovea with overhanging inner retinal tissue.

## Symptoms and clinical findings

Lamellar macular holes are typically stable over prolonged periods. Patients may report a range of visual symptoms and visual acuity can vary from near normal to as poor as 20/400.

## Treatment/prognosis/follow-up

Lamellar macular holes are often stable and of only modest visual impact and therefore observation alone is often the treatment of choice. Surgical intervention with vitrectomy and membrane peeling, especially in the setting of concurrent ERM may be considered. The presence of significant visual impairment or documented progression may favor surgical intervention. Though anatomical improvement following surgery is typical, visual gains are less frequent and typically only modest.

# Further reading

Witkin AJ, Ko TH, Fujimoto JG, et al. Redefining lamellar holes and the vitreomacular interface: an ultrahigh-resolution optical coherence tomography study. Ophthalmology 2006; 113:388–97.

Witkin AJ, Castro LC, Reichel E, et al. Anatomic and visual outcomes of vitrectomy for lamellar macular holes. Ophthalmic Surg Lasers Imaging 2010; 41:418–24.

# 22

# Vitreomacular traction syndrome

## How to approach a patient with a blunted foveal reflex

| Identify the primary pathologic clinical finding(s) | | |
|---|---|---|
| On examination, there is obscuration of the normal foveal reflex but with the absence of a full-thickness defect (**Figure 22.1**). | | |
| **Formulate a differential diagnosis** | | |
| Most likely | Less likely | Least likely |
| • Vitreomacular traction (VMT) syndrome | • Macular hole, pattern dystrophy, macular degeneration | • Cystoid macular edema, epiretinal membrane, photic retinopathy, MacTel type II, cone dystrophy |
| **Query patient history** | | |
| • Are there any visual symptoms such as distorted or decreased visual acuity?<br>• Is there a central scotoma?<br>• Has there been recent ocular surgery?<br>• What is the age of the patient?<br>• Has there been any history of sun-gazing or light toxicity to the retina? | | |
| **Decide on ancillary diagnostic imaging** | | |
| Optical coherence tomography (OCT) is very useful to image the vitreomacular interface and can be diagnostic of numerous conditions within the differential diagnosis. | | |

## Ancillary diagnostic imaging interpretation

### Optical coherence tomography

OCT reveals the presence of VMT and absence of findings consistent with the other potential diagnoses. There is focal VMT with disturbance of the normal foveal indentation (**Figure 22.2**).

## Final diagnosis: vitreomacular traction syndrome

### Epidemiology/etiology

An anomalous posterior vitreous detachment occurs when there is insufficient separation of the posterior hyaloid from the retina. Resultant adhesions between the vitreous and surface of the retina can cause traction-related deformation of the retinal layers, which when occurring in the macula is called VMT. To meet the definition of VMT [as defined by the International Vitreomacular Traction Study Classification System (Duker et al. 2013)], there must be a perifoveal posterior vitreous detachment in combination with anatomical distortion of the macula visible on OCT. This must occur in the absence of a full-thickness retinal defect (macular hole, see Chapter 20). Prior

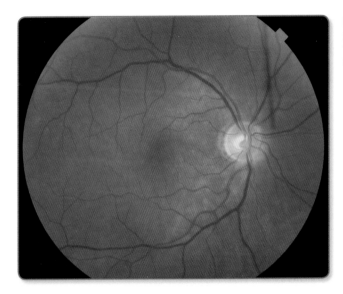

**Figure 22.1** Color fundus photograph of vitreomacular traction. There is disruption of the normal foveal reflex.

to the advent of OCT, this condition was poorly understood and not well described. Historical classification schemes predating OCT and current nomenclature would have considered VMT to be a 'stage 1' or 'impending macular hole.'

## Symptoms and clinical findings

VMT can be asymptomatic and findings on OCT do not always correlate with symptoms. When symptomatic, patients often have distortion of the vision (metamorphopsia) and decreased visual acuity. VMT can be classified as focal (≤1500 μm) or broad (≥1500 μm) based on the OCT appearance, which can be varied. Secondary changes in the macula, which include schisis, macular edema, and generalized thickening may result from the tractional forces that occur in VMT.

## Treatment/prognosis/follow-up

Treatment depends on the presence (and severity) or absence of symptoms. In an asymptomatic patient, observation alone is warranted. In the symptomatic patient, an initial period of observation is generally warranted because some cases will resolve spontaneously (**Figure 22.2d**). In the symptomatic patient that does not self-resolve, treatment is usually indicated. For focal VMT, options include pharmacologic lysis with ocriplasmin (in the absence of concurrent ERM) or surgical elevation of the hyaloid via vitrectomy. For broad VMT, surgical intervention is the only option. Prognosis is generally good. Patients are followed up dependent on severity and whether treatment has been undertaken.

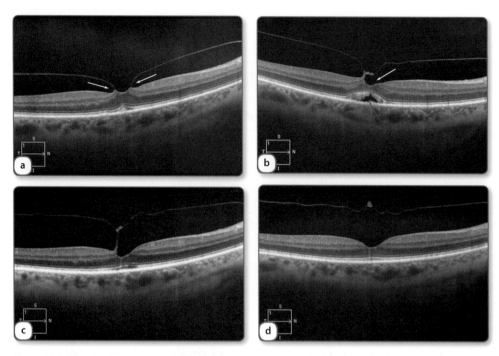

**Figure 22.2** Optical coherence tomography of vitreomacular traction (VMT) syndrome (a–d). (a) Focal VMT with significant distortion of the fovea at presentation. The posterior vitreous is well visualized inserting on both sides of the focal adhesion (arrows). (b) Five months after presentation, there is partial release of the VMT (white arrow) with development of a subfoveal cavity (red arrow). (c) Seven months after presentation, there is continued release of the VMT with resolution of the subfoveal cavity. (d) Fourteen months after presentation, there is spontaneous complete release of the VMT with return of normal foveal architecture.

# Reference

Duker JS, Kaiser PK, Binder S, et al. The international vitreomacular traction study group classification of vitreomacular adhesion, traction, and macular hole. Ophthalmology 2013; 120:2611–19.

# Further reading

Johnson MW. Posterior vitreous detachment: evolution and complications of its early stages. Am J Ophthalmol 2010; 149:371–82.e1.

# 23 | Epiretinal membrane

## How to approach a patient with significant metamorphopsia

| Identify the primary pathologic clinical finding(s) | | |
|---|---|---|
| On examination, there is a visible membrane overlying the surface of the macula associated with retinal striae and dragging of the vasculature (**Figure 23.1**). | | |
| **Formulate a differential diagnosis** | | |
| **Most likely** | **Less likely** | **Least likely** |
| • Epiretinal membrane (ERM), vitreomacular traction | • Lamellar macular hole, full-thickness macular hole | • Macular schisis, cystoid macular edema |
| **Query patient history** | | |
| • Is there metamorphopsia? <br> • Is there micropsia? <br> • Is the visual acuity decreased and by how much? <br> • Is there a central scotoma in the visual field? <br> • Have the symptoms been of gradual or more sudden onset? | | |
| **Decide on ancillary diagnostic imaging** | | |
| Optical coherence tomography (OCT) is the best diagnostic test to confirm the presence of a suspected ERM. OCT will also help to rule out many of the other diagnoses being considered in the differential. FA can identify associated vascular leakage and may be useful if the underlying diagnosis is in question but in general angiography is not necessary. | | |

## Ancillary diagnostic imaging interpretation

### Optical coherence tomography

OCT shows a highly reflective preretinal membrane overlying the surface of the macula (**Figure 23.2**). The underlying macula can have a variable degree of irregularity with a foveal contour that can be nearly normal or completely obscured depending on severity. Other features that may be present include thickening of the retinal layers (best seen on corresponding thickness map), intraretinal cysts, and sometimes subretinal fluid.

## Final diagnosis: ERM

### Epidemiology/etiology

ERMs are composed of fibrous tissue that proliferates on the surface of the macula, between the posterior hyaloid and internal limiting membrane. Contracture of this tissue results in macular distortion with symptoms that typically correlate with the severity of the mechanical effect. There are numerous secondary causes for ERM formation such as retinal tears, intraocular inflammation or infection, prior venous occlusion, and trauma. More commonly, ERMs are thought to be related to residual posterior cortical vitreous that remains on the macular surface following posterior vitreous detachment (vitreoschisis). This residual vitreous provides a scaffold for cellular elements (from the

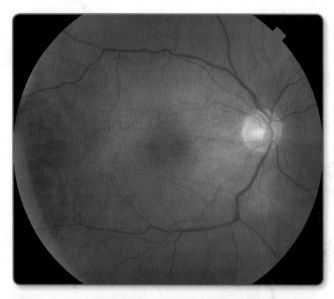

**Figure 23.1** Color photograph of epiretinal membrane. There is an irregular sheen to the surface of the macula with a visible semitranslucent membrane overlying the retinal tissue. Retinal striae are visible, particularly superiorly, and there is mild dragging of the vasculature.

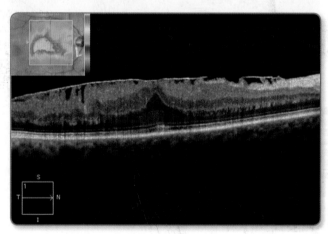

**Figure 23.2** Optical coherence tomography of epiretinal membrane preoperatively (corresponds to Figure 23.1). Typical features include a hyper-reflective membrane overlying the preretinal surface, which represents the epiretinal membrane in cross section. There is a significant increase in macular thickening best visualized on the accompanying thickness map (inset). There is also complete loss of the foveal depression and the retinal surface is jagged.

retina and RPE) to proliferate, which forms the ERM. ERM is a relatively common finding that becomes more prevalent with age.

## Symptoms and clinical findings

Metamorphopsia or distortion of vision is the primary symptom attributed to an ERM and can be significant even in the absence of significant visual acuity impairment. An ERM may also commonly be associated with a variable degree of visual acuity loss. Less common visual symptoms include monocular diplopia and micropsia. Presenting visual acuity can range from 20/20 to as poor as 20/400. An ERM occurs overlying the macula and clinically can be appreciated as a semitranslucent surface membrane with an irregular sheen. Secondary effects due to tractional distortion of the retinal tissue can occasionally

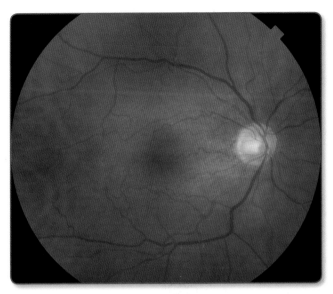

**Figure 23.3** Color photograph of epiretinal membrane postoperatively. One month following vitrectomy with membrane peeling, the macula has a much more normal appearance with significant improvement in all the features depicted in Figure 23.1.

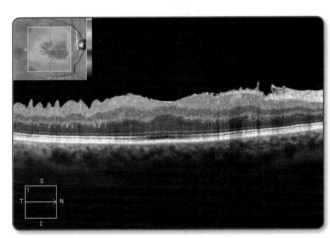

**Figure 23.4** Optical coherence tomography of epiretinal membrane postoperatively (corresponds to Figure 23.3). The overlying epiretinal membrane is noticeably removed from the central macular surface. Retinal thickness has improved somewhat and the foveal depression has also begun to return. Additional improvements would be expected over the ensuing months.

cause a pseudohole appearance, intraretinal hemorrhage, vascular dragging, and even cystoid macular edema. Synonyms for ERM include macular pucker and cellophane maculopathy.

## Treatment/prognosis/follow-up

Without surgical removal, an ERM typically will worsen to a point and then stabilize with a variable effect on vision. Most patients with ERM have minimal symptoms and observation alone is warranted. If visual symptoms are sufficient to warrant surgical intervention, a majority of patients (~75%) will appreciate a two or more line improvement in visual acuity. The improvement is typically slow, occurring over months, even up to a year after surgery (**Figures 23.2** and **23.4**).

## How to approach a patient with a discrete round lesion in the fovea

| Identify the primary pathologic clinical finding(s) | | |
|---|---|---|
| There is a distinct round, reddish defect in the fovea associated with an epiretinal membrane (**Figure 24.1**). | | |
| **Formulate a differential diagnosis** | | |
| **Most likely** | **Less likely** | **Least likely** |
| • Macular pseudohole, full-thickness macular hole | • Lamellar macular hole, vitreomacular traction syndrome | • Cystoid macular edema, macular scar |
| **Query patient history** | | |
| • Is there a central defect in vision (scotoma)?<br>• If there is a visual impairment, how long has this been present for? | | |
| **Decide on ancillary diagnostic imaging** | | |
| Optical coherence tomography (OCT) is the most useful diagnostic test for distinguishing the diagnoses being considered in the differential. | | |

## Ancillary diagnostic imaging interpretation

### Optical coherence tomography

OCT shows the presence of an epiretinal membrane (ERM) with heaping of the central foveal tissue (**Figure 24.2**). A key distinction of macular pseudohole from full-thickness or lamellar macular hole is that there is no loss of foveal tissue in a pseudohole.

## Final diagnosis: macular pseudohole

### Epidemiology/etiology

Macular pseudohole is a clinical diagnosis made at the slit lamp supplemented by confirmatory OCT testing. The presence of an ERM causes contracture of the macula with heaping of tissue toward the center, which results in a clinical appearance that resembles a full-thickness macular hole but with no actual loss of tissue as evidenced by OCT.

### Symptoms and clinical findings

Patients may experience blurring or distortion of vision but a central scotoma should not be present. In mild cases, symptoms may be minimal. The clinical appearance resembles that of a full-thickness macular hole centered within an ERM. Patients should not note a

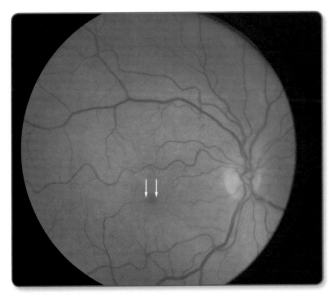

**Figure 24.1** Color photograph of macular pseudohole. There is a distinct, round, reddish apparent defect in the center of the macula surrounded by a mild, diffuse, ERM. Arrows correspond to optical coherence tomography.

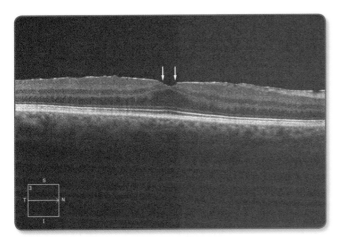

**Figure 24.2** Optical coherence tomography of macular pseudohole. An ERM is present on the surface of the macula causing contracture of the underlying tissue with loss of the typical foveal depression due to heaped up tissue (between arrows), which corresponds to the apparent hole seen clinically. Not that there is no loss of tissue as is seen in lamellar or full-thickness macular holes.

central gap of light when a slit beam is positioned directly over the pseudohole (negative Watzke-Allen sign), which helps distinguish this entity from full-thickness macular hole.

## Treatment/prognosis/follow-up

The need for treatment is based on the degree of symptoms and the impairment that these cause to the patient. Symptoms in the setting of a macular pseudohole are attributable to the concurrent ERM and management is directed toward surgical removal. If symptoms justify treatment, pars plana vitrectomy with epiretinal membrane peeling is the standard approach.

# Posterior vitreous detachment

## How to approach a patient with new onset of photopsias and prominent floater(s) in one eye

| Identify the primary pathologic clinical finding(s) | | |
| --- | --- | --- |
| Examination reveals a prominent circular, c-, or u-shaped vitreous opacity suspended in the vitreous cavity within proximity to the optic nerve (**Figure 25.1**). | | |
| **Formulate a differential diagnosis** | | |
| **Most likely** | **Less likely** | **Least likely** |
| • Acute posterior vitreous detachment, impending/evolving vitreous detachment | • Retinal tear, retinal detachment, ocular migraine | • Intraocular inflammation (uveitis) |
| **Query patient history** | | |
| • Are the photopsias (flashes of light) more prominent in a dark environment or at night?<br>• Was there a shower of floaters that looked like pepper flakes?<br>• Has there been a change in vision or curtain/shade over peripheral vision?<br>• Are the symptoms better, worse, or stable since onset? | | |
| **Decide on ancillary diagnostic imaging** | | |
| A thorough ophthalmic examination including a detailed inspection of the peripheral retina with scleral depression is sufficient to differentiate most of the diagnostic considerations. No ancillary diagnostic testing is required. | | |

## Ancillary diagnostic imaging interpretation

### Optical coherence tomography

Optical coherence tomography (OCT) may be useful in certain clinical scenarios to aid in the diagnosis of a patient with these presenting symptoms. OCT is not typically ordered for the purpose of diagnosing a posterior vitreous detachment (PVD) but can be illustrative for educational purposes. See discussion for more details.

## Final diagnosis: acute posterior vitreous detachment

### Epidemiology/etiology

Vitreous detachment from the retina is an insidious physiological event that takes place over years, culminating in posterior separation of the cortical vitreous from the back wall of the eye or PVD. It is only during this last stage of PVD evolution when symptoms typically occur, coinciding with the clinical appearance of a Weiss ring, which suggests complete vitreopapillary separation. This event is called an acute PVD. The process of PVD is physiologic and age-related in the majority of

# Section 5

# Other macular disorders

# Toxic maculopathy

## How to approach a patient with a bull's-eye maculopathy

| Identify the primary pathologic clinical finding(s) | | |
|---|---|---|
| Clinical examination of the right eye is within normal limits. The left eye demonstrates a very subtle parafoveal ring of atrophy. | | |
| **Formulate a differential diagnosis** | | |
| **Most likely** | **Less likely** | **Least likely** |
| • Hydroxychloroquine (Plaquenil) toxicity | • Cone and cone–rod dystrophy, chloroquine toxicity, macular degeneration | • Benign concentric annular dystrophy, vitelliform macular dystrophy, retinitis pigmentosa |
| **Query patient history** | | |
| • Is there a history of an autoimmune condition?<br>• Does the patient have difficulty reading? Has the patient noted that letters are sometimes slanted or missing? Does the patient have to go back and reread things repeatedly?<br>• Is the patient taking any medicines? For how long? At what dose?<br>• How tall is the patient?<br>• Does the patient have kidney or liver problems?<br>• Is their a family history of similar retinal problems? How is the patient's night vision? | | |
| **Decide on ancillary diagnostic imaging** | | |
| Fundus photography is useful for patient education, but is insensitive as a screening tool for hydroxychloroquine toxicity. Optical coherence tomography (OCT) is instrumental in the early detection of hydroxychloroquine toxicity. Thinning of the outer nuclear layer and attenuation of the parafoveal outer retinal layers are the earliest signs of toxicity. Later findings include the 'flying saucer' sign, which results from relative preservation of central foveal outer retina in the setting of severe parafoveal outer retinal thinning. End-stage OCT appearance consists of RPE migration and diffuse outer retinal atrophy that can mimic end-stage macular degeneration or a severe cone or cone–rod dystrophy. 10-2 visual fields are another useful adjunct for screening. Of note, there is a small subset of patients who have normal SD-OCT findings but reliably demonstrate ring scotomas on central field testing. Multifocal ERG testing can also detect subtle toxicity, but this test is mainly limited to research settings. Fluorescein angiography and fundus autofluorescence detect toxicity at relatively later stages and, as such, have lesser utility as a screening entity. Color vision testing or home Amsler grid testing are no longer considered reliable screening tools for hydroxychloroquine toxicity. | | |

## Ancillary diagnostic imaging interpretation

### Color photography

Color photography reveals a very subtle circular area of atrophy in the left eye. The right eye appears normal (**Figure 30.1**).

### Optical coherence tomography

The infrared images demonstrate a bull's-eye pattern in both eyes. The color maps appear more bluish than normal, indicative of retinal thinning.

Horizontal cuts through the right eye reveal severe paracentral outer retinal atrophy. There is an early 'flying saucer' or 'sombrero' sign. The outer nuclear layers are attenuated. The left eye has a similar appearance with collapse and atrophy of the paracentral outer retina (**Figure 30.2**).

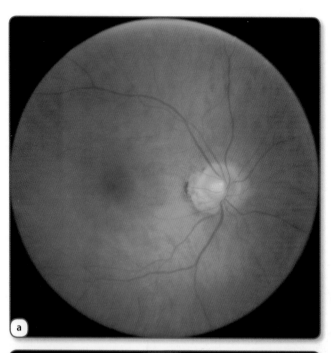

**Figure 30.1** Color photographs of the (a) right and (b) left eyes. There is no clear abnormality in the right eye. The left eye has a subtle ring of RPE atrophy.

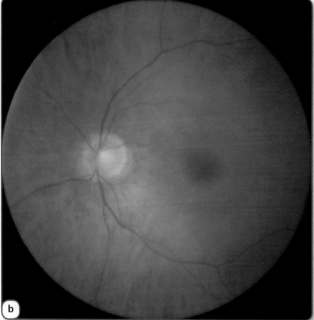

## Humphrey visual field testing

A 24-2 study demonstrates a central scotoma in both eyes. Two years after drug cessation, a 10-2 illustrates persistent ring scotomas (**Figure 30.3**).

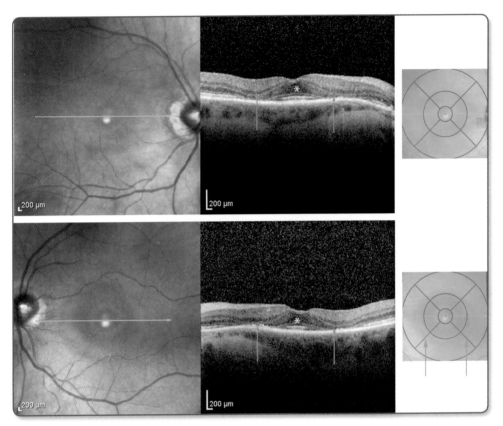

**Figure 30.2** Optical coherence tomography of both eyes. Infrared images and color maps demonstrate a bull's-eye pattern in both eyes, best illustrated in the left eye (blue arrows). Serial horizontal slices demonstrate the 'flying saucer' sign (asterisk). There is loss of all outer retina bands and outer nuclear thinning on both sides of the fovea (red arrows).

# Final diagnosis: hydroxychloroquine toxicity

## Epidemiology/etiology

Hydroxychloroquine is an effective and relatively safe medicine used for many rheumatologic disorders, including rheumatoid arthritis and lupus. The likelihood of retinal toxicity from hydroxychloroquine has historically felt to be low. However, with the widespread adoption of spectral-domain OCT, it is becoming increasingly apparent that the prevalence of hydroxychloroquine toxicity is much higher than initially thought.

The risk of toxicity is directly related to daily dose and cumulative lifetime dose. Dosing should be based on ideal body weight. Therefore, only women taller than 5'6" should consume 400 mg daily. Women shorter than 5'0" should be on 200 mg daily. The dose should be reduced in patients with renal or liver compromise. Once appropriately dosed patients reach approximately 1000 g of consumption, they are felt to be at a higher risk of toxicity.

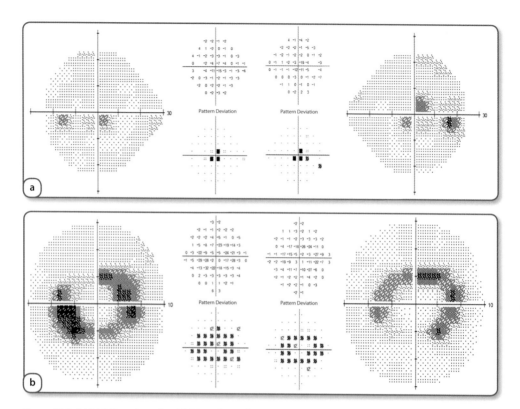

**Figure 30.3** (a) 24-2 Humphrey visual fields performed at presentation demonstrate paracentral scotomas. The hydroxychloroquine was stopped. (b) Two years after drug cessation, 10-2 Humphrey visual fields show persistent ring scotomas.

Hydroxychloroquine binds to melanin in the RPE, where, over time, it leads to RPE cell death and atrophy. Ultimately, this leads to irreversible photoreceptor loss.

## Symptoms and clinical findings

Early in the disease process, patients may be asymptomatic and the fundus appears entirely normal. As exposure to the drug increases, symptoms such as flashing lights, difficulty reading, and metamorphopsia may develop and clinical examination can demonstrate loss of the foveal light reflex or mild RPE mottling and stippling. Without cessation of the drug, patients begin to notice color vision abnormalities and blurred vision at all distances. A bull's-eye maculopathy may ultimately develop with the appearance of concentric rings of hyper- and hypo-pigmentation around the fovea. End-stage hydroxychloroquine toxicity can result in legal blindness.

## Treatment/prognosis/follow-up

The American Academy of Ophthalmology has published rigorous and evidence-based guidelines for hydroxychloroquine screening.

All patients should have a baseline examination to assess for pre-existing retinal pathology and to educate them about the risks of long term hydroxychloroquine use. After year five of drug consumption, yearly visits with OCT and 10-2 testing are then recommended. Patients with liver or kidney disease should be considered high risk and screened yearly after the baseline examination.

Once any sign of hydroxychloroquine toxicity is detected, the prescribing physician should be consulted and the medication stopped. Toxicity can progress for years despite drug cessation. The earlier the medication is stopped, the better the ultimate outcome for the patient.

## Further reading

Marmor MF. Comparison of screening procedures in hydroxychloroquine toxicity. Arch Ophthalmol 2012; 130:461–9.

Marmor MF, Kellner U, Lai TY, et al. Revised recommendations on screening for chloroquine and hydroxychloroquine retinopathy. Ophthalmology 2011; 118:415–22.

Marmor MF, Melles RB. Disparity between visual fields and optical coherence tomography in hydroxychloroquine retinopathy. Ophthalmology 2014;121:1257-1262.

## How to approach a patient with focal foveal abnormalities

| Identify the primary pathologic clinical finding(s) | | |
|---|---|---|
| Clinical examination of the right eye is within normal limits. The left eye demonstrates a discreet oval-shaped yellow lesion within the fovea. | | |
| **Formulate a differential diagnosis** | | |
| **Most likely** | **Less likely** | **Least likely** |
| • Laser-induced maculopathy | • Solar or solar eclipse retinopathy, welder's retinopathy, Alkyl nitrate abuse, whiplash retinopathy | • Impending macular hole, foveolar vitreomacular traction, tamoxifen retinopathy |
| **Query patient history** | | |
| • Does the patient have a history of sun gazing, laser pointer exposure or welding?<br>• Does the patient take any medications? | | |
| **Decide on ancillary diagnostic imaging** | | |
| Fundus photography is useful to demonstrate the lesion and for patient education. Optical coherence tomography (OCT) can best identify the location and extent of foveal abnormality. OCT can also help differentiate between the various diagnostic possibilities; for instance, vitreomacular traction can readily be diagnosed. Furthermore, it is the best device for tracking subtle outer retinal changes over time. Fluorescein angiography, indocyanine green and fundus autofluorescence are less valuable in the management of these disorders. | | |

## Ancillary diagnostic imaging interpretation

### Color photography

Color photography of the right eye is within normal limits. The left eye has a yellowish plaque located within the fovea. There is a small orange ring surrounding the lesion. There is no associated hemorrhage (**Figure 31.1**).

### Optical coherence tomography

Ultrahigh resolution OCT demonstrates a full-thickness isoreflective lesion traversing the fovea. The outer retinal and retinal pigment epithelium bands are disrupted within the foveal area (**Figure 31.2a**). There a small amount of subretinal fluid.

One month after presentation, a focal outer retinal defect remains. There is some pigment migration within the wedge-shaped outer retinal defect (**Figure 31.2b**).

### Fluorescein angiography

Early phase angiograph shows a subtle hyperfluorescent ring within the fovea. The borders of the lesion stain during the study, and there is mild leakage at the nasal border (**Figure 31.3**).

# How to approach a patient with new onset of a shower of floaters

| Identify the primary pathologic clinical finding(s) | | |
|---|---|---|
| There is an elevated retinal flap on the edge of a full-thickness retinal defect located in the peripheral fundus. | | |
| **Formulate a differential diagnosis** | | |
| **Most likely** | **Less likely** | **Least likely** |
| • Retinal tear, retinal detachment | • Posterior vitreous detachment, vitreous hemorrhage | • Uveitis |
| **Query patient history** | | |
| • When did the symptoms start?<br>• Are there associated photopsias, particularly in a dark environment or at night?<br>• Is there an associated visual impairment of visual field cut?<br>• What is the age of the patient?<br>• Was there any recent trauma? | | |
| **Decide on ancillary diagnostic imaging** | | |
| A careful examination of the involved eye with indirect ophthalmoscopy and 360° scleral depression is the most important method to evaluate the entities being considered in the differential diagnosis. If significant media opacity is present (i.e. from vitreous hemorrhage), B-scan ultrasound should be performed to evaluate for retinal tear or detachment. | | |

## Ancillary diagnostic imaging interpretation

None.

## Final diagnosis: retinal tear

### Epidemiology/etiology

Retinal tears typically occur in the far peripheral retina near the vitreous base insertion and are a result of pathophysiologic vitreoretinal traction in this location, often occurring concurrent with an acute posterior vitreous detachment. Due to anatomical variations in vitreous base insertions, tears can occur anywhere from the mid-periphery anteriorly to the ora serrata. Acute retinal tears are often horseshoe in their configuration due to the location of overlying vitreoretinal tractional forces (**Figure 32.1**), hence the term horseshoe retinal tear. Risk factors include increasing age, high myopia, lattice degeneration, and trauma.

### Symptoms and clinical findings

A shower of black floaters is the typical symptom associated with the onset of an acute retinal tear. Other symptoms may include photopsias

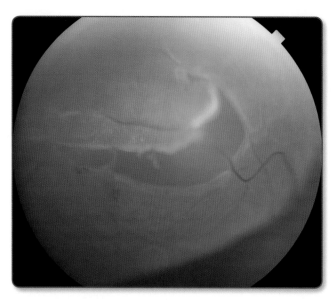

**Figure 32.1** Color photograph of a horseshoe retinal tear. There is an acute retinal tear with characteristic horseshoe configuration. There is also an associated retinal detachment and two bridging retinal blood vessels present.

## Differential diagnosis in a patient with new floaters

Retinal tear
Retinal detachment
Posterior vitreous detachment
Vitreous hemorrhage
Uveitis

and, possibly, decreased visual acuity if associated with vitreous hemorrhage. If a visual field defect is present, a concurrent retinal detachment should be suspected. In a retinal tear that has been present for more than a few months, pigment deposits surrounding the margins may develop due to natural chorioretinal adhesions. Persistent vitreous traction may lead to the flap of the tear disinserting so that it is free floating in the vitreous cavity, leaving an operculated retinal hole.

### Treatment/prognosis/follow-up

Prompt treatment (retinopexy) for an acute, symptomatic retinal tear is recommended with laser photocoagulation to surround the tear or cryotherapy to the entire region of the tear. Treatment significantly reduces the risk of subsequent retinal detachment and vision loss. If a retinal tear is asymptomatic and has features of chronicity, such as surrounding pigment demarcation, observation may be appropriate.

## How to approach a patient with a peripheral visual field defect, new floaters, and decreased vision

| Identify the primary pathologic clinical finding(s) | | |
|---|---|---|
| Examination of the retina reveals a retinal tear associated with an area of retinal elevation with underlying clear fluid. An associated posterior vitreous detachment is often present (**Figure 33.1**). | | |
| **Formulate a differential diagnosis** | | |
| **Most likely** | **Less likely** | **Least likely** |
| • Rhegmatogenous retinal detachment, retinoschisis | • Retinal tear, tractional retinal detachment, exudative retinal detachment | • Choroidal detachment, choroidal infiltration or tumor, posterior scleritis |
| **Query patient history** | | |
| • Did the patient experience the sudden onset of dark floaters in a single eye?<br>• Does the patient notice a dark shadow in their peripheral vision that is enlarging towards the center of their vision?<br>• Is the patient highly myopic?<br>• Has the patient had any recent significant ocular trauma? | | |
| **Decide on ancillary diagnostic imaging** | | |
| The diagnosis can usually be made clinically based on careful fundoscopic examination. In cases where retinoschisis and rhegmatogenous retinal detachment are both being considered, optical coherence tomography (OCT) is invaluable in differentiating the two. B-scan ultrasound may also occasionally be needed to confirm the diagnosis, especially if significant media opacity is present. | | |

## Ancillary diagnostic imaging interpretation

### Optical coherence tomography

OCT is useful in the setting of known rhegmatogenous retinal detachment to evaluate for the presence of subretinal fluid in the macula, which may be subtle or imperceptible clinically, if shallow (**Figure 33.2**). OCT is also valuable in assessing the peripheral retinal to differentiate retinal detachment from retinoschisis, which can sometimes be difficult to distinguish clinically.

## Final diagnosis: rhegmatogenous retinal detachment

### Epidemiology/etiology

There are three types of retinal detachment: rhegmatogenous, tractional, and serous (exudative). Rhegmatogenous detachments are the most common and occur due to the transit of liquefied vitreous fluid into the subretinal space via a retinal defect such as a hole or tear. Tractional detachments occur as a result of abnormal vitreous fibrous proliferation with underlying retinal traction, most commonly in the setting of proliferative diabetic retinopathy. Serous or exudative retinal detachments are the least common of the three types and occur secondary to leakage related to ocular tumors and, rarely, due

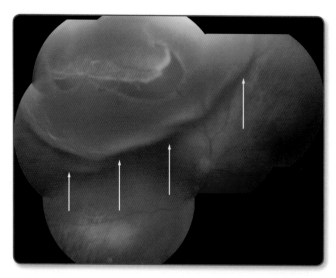

**Figure 33.1** Color photograph in retinal detachment. There is a large retinal tear associated with a bullous superotemporal rhegmatogenous macula-off retinal detachment (margins illustrated by arrows).

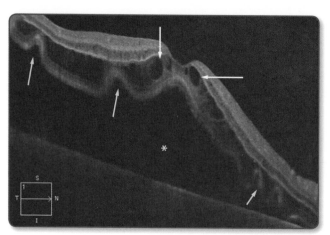

**Figure 33.2** Optical coherence tomography (OCT) in retinal detachment. OCT reveals subretinal fluid in the macula (asterisk), indicating this is a macula-off retinal detachment. Characteristic retinal folds are present (yellow arrows) in addition to cystoid macular edema (white arrows), which is not uncommonly associated with retinal detachments.

to systemic medical conditions. Rhegmatogenous detachments are the most common and occur due to the transit of liquefied vitreous fluid into the subretinal space via retinal defect such as a hole or tear.

## Symptoms and clinical findings

A defect in the peripheral vision is almost always present but sometimes has to be brought to the patients' attention. The visual field defect would be expected in the opposite quadrant as the detached area. If the macula is affected, central visual acuity will be decreased. Common associated symptoms include new floaters and/or photopsias. A rhegmatogenous retinal detachment appears as an elevated area of retina that begins in the periphery and spreads towards the posterior pole (**Figure 33.1**).

## Treatment/prognosis/follow-up

Rhegmatogenous retinal detachments can be managed by various methods depending on the location, severity, and other preoperative factors. These methods include laser retinopexy (reserved for small, typically asymptomatic detachments), pneumatic retinopexy, scleral buckling, vitrectomy, or combined scleral buckle and vitrectomy. An associated culprit retinal tear should be identified to assist in determining the optimal treatment approach. With the exception of laser retinopexy, which walls off the detachment and prevents extension, the other methods for repair strive to achieve resolution of the subretinal fluid and sealing of the culprit retinal tear(s) or hole(s) to prevent reaccumulation of subretinal fluid. Retinal detachments need to be repaired in a timely manner to maximize anatomical and visual outcomes, particularly in macula-on detachments when the macula is imminently threatened from detaching. If the macula is detached preoperatively, the ultimate visual prognosis is less favorable.

## How to approach a patient with linear peripheral retinal pigmentation

| Identify the primary pathologic clinical finding(s) | | |
|---|---|---|
| Indirect ophthalmoscopy reveals flat, linear, pigmented areas in the retinal periphery arranged in patches running roughly parallel to the ora serrata. | | |
| **Formulate a differential diagnosis** | | |
| **Most likely** | **Less likely** | **Least likely** |
| • Lattice degeneration | • Chorioretinal scar, reticular degeneration, cobblestone degeneration | • White without pressure |
| **Query patient history** | | |
| • Has there been a history of retinal detachment in the fellow eye?<br>• What is the patients' refractive error?<br>• How old is the patient? | | |
| **Decide on ancillary diagnostic imaging** | | |
| The diagnosis of lattice degeneration is made on clinical grounds. | | |

## Ancillary diagnostic imaging interpretation

None.

## Final diagnosis: lattice degeneration

### Epidemiology/etiology

Lattice degeneration is a common peripheral retinal abnormality that is seen in up to 10% of the general population. Patients with this condition are at higher risk for retinal tears and detachment than those without the condition, although the risk is still low. Overlying areas of lattice degeneration, the vitreous is liquefied and adherent along the edges, where there is a propensity to develop retinal tears, particularly during posterior vitreous detachment. Patients with myopia are more likely to have lattice degeneration.

### Symptoms and clinical findings

Most patients with lattice degeneration are asymptomatic and, therefore, the diagnosis is typically made during routine fundoscopy. In the presence of associated retinal traction, retinal tear, or detachment there may be symptoms such as photopsias and floaters. The appearance and severity of lattice degeneration can be varied. There can be a single, small isolated patch in one eye in mild cases or there can be many, large patches affecting both eyes in more severe cases. Lattice characteristically appears as a linear patch of pigmentation within the retina along with sclerotic vessels arranged in a lattice-like arrangement (**Figure 34.1**), which affords lattice degeneration its name. Atrophic holes within areas of lattice degeneration are common (**Figure 34.2**).

## Treatment/prognosis/follow-up

No treatment is typically necessary or recommended for isolated lattice degeneration. In the setting of lattice degeneration in the fellow eye of a patient who has had a prior retinal detachment, prophylactic laser retinopexy may provide a modest reduction of risk for subsequent retinal detachment, although this effect may be lost in eyes with extensive lattice or high myopia. Prophylactic retinopexy is generally recommended for lattice degeneration in the setting of retinal tear or subclinical retinal detachment. Patients with lattice degeneration should be educated about the symptoms of retinal tear and detachment and instructed to seek timely care should such symptoms develop.

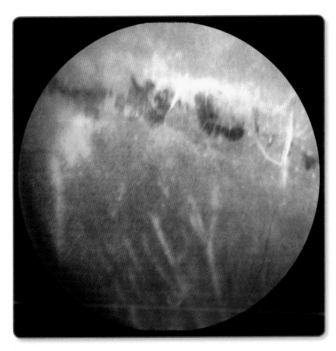

**Figure 34.1** Typical lattice degeneration. This photograph demonstrates a linear pattern of lattice degeneration in the peripheral retina with characteristic scattered dark pigmentation and sclerotic vessels in a lattice-like arrangement. By courtesy of Larry Halperin, MD, Boca Raton, Florida. USA.

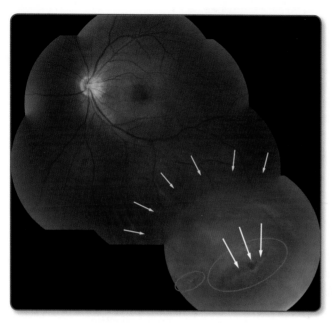

**Figure 34.2** Lattice degeneration and atrophic holes. This photograph demonstrates two separate patches of lattice degeneration (red circles), which have caused a retinal detachment (yellow arrows). The larger patch of lattice degeneration has atrophic holes within it (white arrows), which provided the route for the retinal detachment to form.

# Further reading

Folk JC, Arrindell EL, Klugman MR. The fellow eye of patients with phakic lattice retinal detachment. Ophthalmology 1989; 96:72–9.

# Section 7

# Infectious uveitis

# How to approach a patient with focal retinitis

| Identify the primary pathologic clinical finding(s) | | |
|---|---|---|
| There is a white patch of retinitis just temporal to the fovea in the left eye. The borders of the lesion are indistinct. | | |
| **Formulate a differential diagnosis** | | |
| **Most likely** | **Less likely** | **Least likely** |
| • Ocular toxoplasmosis | • Cat-Scratch disease, intraocular tuberculosis, sarcoidosis | • Progressive outer retinal necrosis, *Candida, Aspergillus,* syphilis |
| **Query patient history** | | |
| • Where is the patient from? South America?<br>• Has the patient travelled internationally?<br>• Has the patient eaten undercooked meat?<br>• Is the patient febrile, have any recent weight loss or night sweats?<br>• Does the patient have any recent contact with cats?<br>• Does the patient have a history of cold sores or genital herpes?<br>• Is the patient immunocompromised? | | |
| **Decide on ancillary diagnostic imaging** | | |
| Fundus photography is useful to document the extent of the process and for patient education. Furthermore, serial photography can help clinicians assess the response to treatment. Optical coherence tomography may demonstrate the depth of retinal infiltration and, as time passes, the degree of irreversible retinal damage. Fluorescein angiography may reveal vasculitis, help to differentiate between the different diagnostic possibilities, and aid in treatment decisions. | | |

# Ancillary diagnostic imaging interpretation

## Color photography

The media is slightly cloudy, likely from vitreous inflammation (**Figure 35.1a**). The retinal vessels are within normal limits. There is a white intraretinal lesion just temporal to the fovea. The borders are fuzzy. Incidentally, there is a large choroidal nevus in the far temporal macula.

## Red-free photography

Red-free images clearly define the extent of the lesion (**Figure 35.1b**).

## Optical coherence tomography

The color map reveals an area of thickening superior-temporal to the fovea. Horizontal B scan through the fovea confirms the irregular thickening (**Figure 35.2**). The inner retina is more hyper-reflective than normal and there is posterior shadowing behind the lesion.

## Fluorescein angiography

Early frames reveal an irregularly angled foveal avascular zone. As the study progresses, there is mild, patchy nonspecific hyperfluorescence in the area around the lesion. Neither papillitis nor vasculitis is noted (**Figure 35.3**).

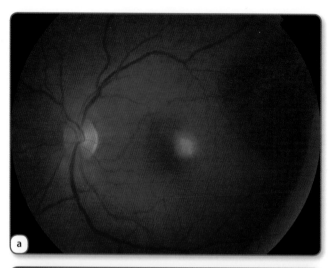

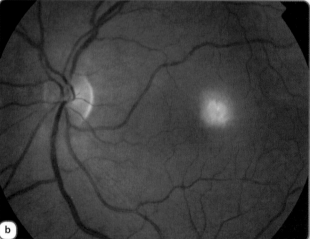

**Figure 35.1** Color (a) and red-free (b) photographs of the left eye. A fluffy white patch of retinitis is seen just temporal to the fovea. There is no vascular sheathing or evident papillitis. A medium size choroidal nevus is present. By courtesy of Caroline Baumal, MD, Boston, MA, USA.

# Final diagnosis: primary ocular toxoplasmosis

## Epidemiology/etiology

*Toxoplasma gondii* is an obligatory intracellular parasite that is the most common cause of posterior uveitis in the United States and in the world. In immunocompromised patients, it is the second most frequent cause of posterior uveitis, next to cytomegalovirus.

Although most active cases represent reactivation of congenital toxoplasmosis, it is becoming increasingly evident that primary acquired infections occur more often than previously thought.

## Symptoms and clinical findings

Affected patients present with blurred vision and floaters and may be referred with the presumed diagnosis of posterior vitreous detachment.

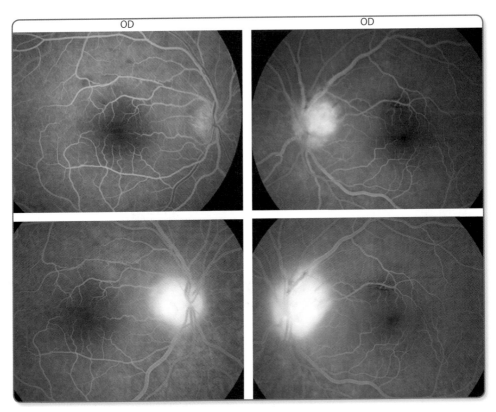

**Figure 36.4** Early (a) and late (b) angiographic images of the right and left eyes. The nerves leak extensively. There are small scattered areas of hypofluorescence, which is the result of blockage by small hemorrhages. There is mild late macular hyperfluorescence, left eye greater than right. By courtesy of Terry Hunter, MD, Oakland, CA, USA.

main findings consist of optic disc edema with peripapillary subretinal fluid. Focal areas of chorioretinitis may be seen in the macula or periphery. As time progresses, intraretinal fluid resorbs and lipid exudates precipitate into Henle's layer. This leads to the appearance of a macular star.

## Treatment/prognosis/follow-up

Laboratory and radiographic evaluation should be guided by clinical history and suspicion (see Box).

Most patients will improve without intervention. That being said, most clinicians will begin antibiotics in hopes of hastening resolution of the disease. Numerous different regiments have been proposed, including azithromycin, doxycycline, rifampin, and erythromycin. Oral steroids may be used as an adjuvant to antimicrobial therapy.

The prognosis for most patients is generally good with a return to baseline visual acuity. There may be mild residual field defect and corresponding sector optic disc pallor.

## Baseline workup for neuroretinitis

*Bartonella* titers: IgM and IgG
RPR and FTA-ABS
Lyme serology
ACE and lysozyme
PPD
Chest X-ray

## Further reading

Ormerod LD, Skolnick KA, Menosky MM, et al. Retinal and choroidal manifestations of cat-scratch disease. Ophthalmology 1998; 105:1024–31.

Reed JB, Scales DK, Wong MT, et al. Bartonella henselae neuroretinitis in cat scratch disease: diagnosis, management, and sequelae. Ophthalmology 1998; 105:459–66.

## How to approach a patient with a hemorrhagic retinitis

| Identify the primary pathologic clinical finding(s) | | |
|---|---|---|
| The panoramic photograph shows perivascular retinal whitening along the inferior arcade out to the periphery. Note the areas of intraretinal hemorrhage. There is also a smaller patch of hemorrhagic retinitis in the superior arcade. | | |
| **Formulate a differential diagnosis** | | |
| Most likely | Less likely | Least likely |
| • Cytomegalovirus (CMV) retinitis | • Acute retinal necrosis, toxoplasmosis, syphilis, tuberculosis, idiopathic frosted branch angiitis | • Sarcoidosis, Behçet's disease, Eales' disease, branch retinal vein occlusion, lymphoma |
| **Query patient history** | | |
| • Does the patient have a history of immunocompromise such as infection with HIV, history of transplant or cancer? <br> • Does the patient have a history of unprotected sex or intravenous drug use? <br> • Does the patient have a history of fever, weight loss or night sweats? <br> • Does the patient have a history of oral or genital herpes? | | |
| **Decide on ancillary diagnostic imaging** | | |
| Fundus photography is helpful to document the extent of retinitis and also for patient education. Serial photographs can help clinicians assess progression or response to treatment, and is often more sensitive than clinical examination. Optical coherence tomography can demonstrate the degree of macular involvement, if applicable. Fluorescein angiography may help if the diagnosis is uncertain, and can also facilitate delineation of the areas of retinitis. | | |

## Ancillary diagnostic imaging interpretation

### Color photography

The media is slightly cloudy from vitreous inflammation. There is a small patch of retinitis along the superior arcade with associated hemorrhage. There is a substantial area of necrosis with intraretinal hemorrhage along the inferior arcade. The retinitis spreads past the horizontal midline. Some gap areas are noted within this region of retinitis. There is a large area of retina and retinal pigment epithelial atrophy in the inferotemporal fundus, apparently formed in the 'wake' of progressive retinitis (**Figure 37.1**).

### Fluorescein angiography

An early wide-field image demonstrates hypofluorescence in the area of peripheral retinitis from incomplete retinal perfusion. There may also be a component of blocking from infected, ischemic retina. Late imaging demonstrates hyperfluorescence due to staining and leakage from infected retinal vessels. The optic nerve appears unaffected (**Figure 37.2**).

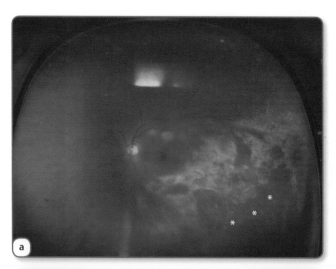

**Figure 37.1** Wide-field color photograph (a) of the left eye in a patient with CMV retinitis. There is a large swath of retinitis following the inferior arcade and crossing the midline. It is encroaching on the macula. There are a few skip areas. There is a large area of retinal and RPE atrophy in its wake (asterisks). An image focused on the posterior pole (b) demonstrates a satellite lesion at the superior arcade as (blue arrow). There is a leading edge of hemorrhage as well at the inferior arcade (red arrow).

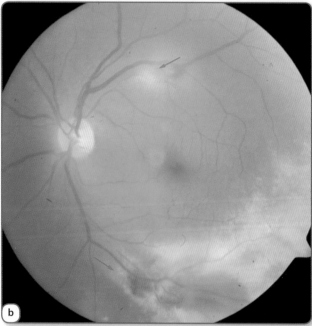

# Final diagnosis: CMV retinitis

## Epidemiology/etiology

CMV retinitis is the most common opportunistic ocular infection and is the leading cause of visual loss in patients with AIDS. CMV retinitis is a marker of significant immune deficiency and thus considered an AIDS-defining illness. Patients usually have a CD4 count <50 cells/mm$^3$, although it can be seen with higher CD4 counts.

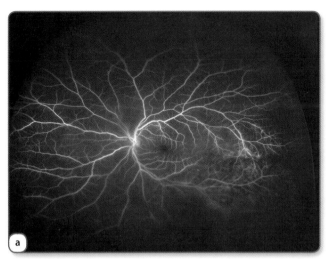

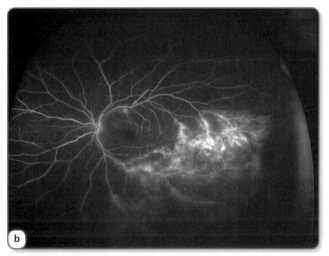

**Figure 37.2** Early (a) and late (b) angiographic images. There is significant late hyperfluorescence from leakage and staining of infiltrated retinal blood vessels. There is also a small area of fluorescence in the superior arcade (blue arrow).

## Symptoms and clinical findings

Small peripheral lesions resembling hemorrhagic cotton-wool spots may be asymptomatic. Patients with posterior lesions involving the macula or optic nerve or those associated with significant vitritis may present with severely decreased vision and visual field defects.

Patches of necrotizing retinitis can be of any size and may be multifocal and bilateral. The disease slowly progresses along retinal blood vessels with areas of confluent retinal whitening and intraretinal hemorrhage. An active leading edge of hemorrhage ('brushfire') may be seen. There is usually only mild vitreous inflammatory response, although it can be more significant in those with higher CD4 counts.

There are alternative appearances of CMV retinitis. It can also present with a granular morphology consisting of a central atrophic area surrounded by punctate white satellite lesions without hemorrhage. A frosted branch angiitis with diffuse vascular sheathing may also be seen.

Zonal atrophy and RPE hyperpigmentation usually appear as the retinitis resolves. Rhegmatogenous retinal detachment is not uncommon and is especially prevalent in myopic patients and those with peripheral pathology.

Diagnosis is typically based on clinical examination and is supported by response to anti-CMV therapy. Blood and urine cultures may also be positive but are relatively nonspecific. Aqueous or vitreous sampling for PCR testing is quite specific and helpful in establishing the diagnosis. When all laboratory testing is equivocal and the diagnosis remains elusive, chorioretinal biopsy may be required.

## Treatment/prognosis/follow-up

Aggressive treatment is required to prevent severe visual loss and treat the underlying infection. The primary medications used to treat CMV retinitis are intravenous ganciclovir, foscarnet, and cidofovir. Oral valganciclovir has also been demonstrated to have potent antiviral properties, as it attains intraocular concentrations that rival intravenous therapy. And oral therapy permits outpatient management of CMV retinitis. Intravitreal ganciclovir (2 mg/0.1 mL) and foscarnet (2.4 mg/0.1 mL) are attractive alternatives, as they deliver high concentrations of antivirals to the retina while avoiding the side effects of systemic therapy. Treatment with all antiviral agents includes an induction phase followed by a maintenance phase to prevent relapse.

In those cases where the presence of CMV retinitis leads to a diagnosis of AIDS, treatment with HAART should also be instituted. Treatment with HAART allows for CD4 counts to rise and decreases viral load, both of which are associated with functional immune recovery.

Immune recovery uveitis may also be seen after initiation of treatment for CMV retinitis. It presents with anterior uveitis, vitritis, and cystoid macular edema and is thought to be a late response to viral antigens. It usually responds well to topical or subtenon's corticosteroids.

## Further reading

Martin DF, Sierra-Madero J, Walmsley S. A controlled trial of valganciclovir as induction therapy for cytomegalovirus retinitis. N Engl J Med 2002; 346:1119–26.

# Acute retinal necrosis

## How to approach a patient with severe intraocular inflammation and peripheral retinal whitening

| Identify the primary pathologic clinical finding(s) | | |
|---|---|---|
| The montage photograph demonstrates fluffy-appearing retinal whitening inferiorly. Peripheral arteries seem to be absent and the veins appear pruned and irregularly filled. There are large dot blot hemorrhages in the periphery. Fresh panretinal photocoagulation (PRP) scars are present (**Figure 38.1a**). | | |
| **Formulate a differential diagnosis** | | |
| **Most likely** | **Less likely** | **Least likely** |
| • Acute retinal necrosis | • Toxoplasmosis, CMV retinitis, intraocular tuberculosis | • Sarcoidosis, Behçet's disease, syphilis, Eales' disease, proliferative diabetic retinopathy with intravitreal Kenalog, ocular ischemic syndrome |
| **Query patient history** | | |
| • Is the patient having fevers, chills or night sweats?<br>• Does the patient have a facial rash or any tingling or burning sensation on the scalp or forehead?<br>• Does the patient have a history of oral or genital herpes?<br>• Is the patient immunocompromised? | | |
| **Decide on ancillary diagnostic imaging** | | |
| Fundus photography is useful to document the extent of the process and for patient education. Furthermore, serial photography can help clinicians assess the response to treatment. Optical coherence tomography may demonstrate inner retinal ischemia, retinal edema, and/or subretinal fluid. Fluorescein angiography may reveal occlusive vasculitis and can help to differentiate between the different diagnostic possibilities. | | |

## Ancillary diagnostic imaging interpretation

### Color photography

The media is slightly cloudy, likely from vitreous inflammation. The retinal arteries are attenuated and thready. The veins are sheathed. Temporal to the fovea, there is retinal whitening with scattered intraretinal hemorrhages. In this area, the vessels are pruned (**Figure 38.1a**). The montage shows a triangular area of heavy retinal whitening inferiorly with satellite lesions encroaching toward the inferior arcade. The retinal arteries are missing peripherally, and the veins are distinctly abnormal in color and caliber. Fresh PRP scars are found 360 and posterior to the area of retinal whitening (**Figure 38.1 a,b**).

### Red-free photography

Red-free images clearly demonstrate the vascular abnormalities. There is severe pruning of the small- and medium-sized retinal vessels (**Figure 38.1c**).

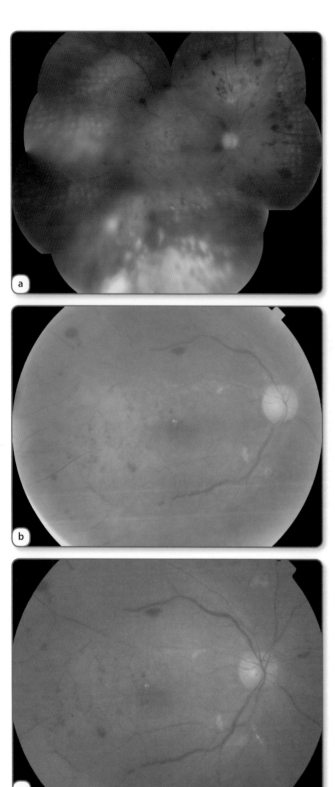

**Figure 38.1** Color (a, b) and red-free (c) images of the right eye. There is active retinitis visible as retinal whitening, scattered intraretinal hemorrhage, and retinal vascular disruption. The PRP has been placed. By courtesy of Caroline Baumal, MD, Boston, MA, USA.

## Optical coherence tomography

A horizontal cross section demonstrates mild intraretinal fluid. Temporally, there are hyper-reflective bands in the inner retina, which is highly suggestive of inner retinal ischemia (**Figure 38.2**).

## Fluorescein angiography

Early frames demonstrate early retinal arterial and venous occlusion, consistent with a necrotizing obliterative angiopathy (**Figure 38.3**). Medium and small vessels do not fill past the arcades. A late image shows moderate macular leakage, vessel, and nerve staining.

# Final diagnosis: acute retinal necrosis

## Epidemiology/etiology

Acute retinal necrosis (ARN) is a rare, severe condition that typically affects middle-aged adults. Unlike other infectious retinopathies, it

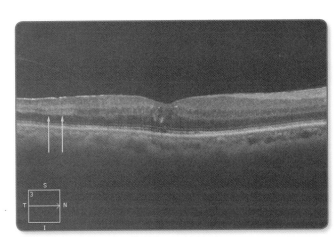

**Figure 38.2** Optical coherence tomography of the right eye. Note the hyperreflective bands (blue arrows) within the inner nuclear layer, which is suggestive of deep capillary ischemia. By courtesy of Caroline Baumal, MD, Boston, MA, USA.

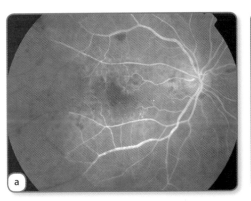
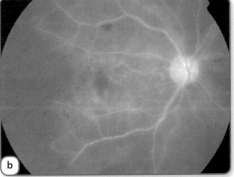

**Figure 38.3** Angiographic images of the right eye demonstrate arterial and venous occlusive disease causing an enlarged foveal avascular zone. By courtesy of Caroline Baumal, MD, Boston, MA, USA.

more often affects immunocompetent patients. Though nearly all members of the herpes virus family have been implicated, the most common pathogens are HSV-1, HSV-2, and VZV.

## Symptoms and clinical findings

Affected patients present with a painful, light sensitive, red eye with poor vision. They may exhibit signs of past or present shingles infection. Examination of the anterior segment can demonstrate a herpetic keratitis, episcleritis, or scleritis. Anterior chamber inflammation is

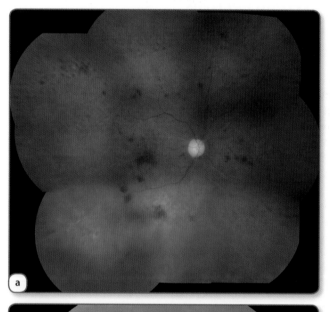

**Figure 38.4** After therapy (a), the retinitis has resolved. Unfortunately, the patient ultimately developed a retinal detachment (b). By courtesy of Caroline Baumal, MD, Boston, MA, USA.

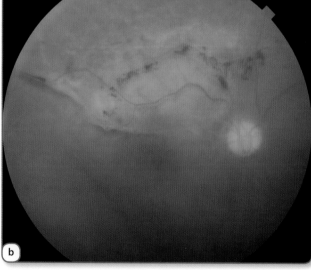

typically severe, with either granulomatous or nongranulomatous keratitic precipitates.

Posterior segment findings have been defined by the American Uveitis Society. Common clinical characteristics include one or more peripheral areas of retinal necrosis with discrete borders, rapid circumferential progression in the absence of appropriate treatment, and an occlusive arterial vasculopathy. A papillitis may also be seen.

## Treatment/prognosis/follow-up

If ARN is suspected, aggressive therapy with antivirals is crucial to prevent progression of the retinitis and to protect the fellow eye that can be involved in a minority of cases. Treatment should be instituted immediately and in most instances should not be delayed until the results of laboratory and aqueous PCR testing become available.

Outpatient management of ARN has become more feasible with the development of newer and more bioavailable forms of acyclovir, such as valacyclovir and famciclovir. These oral agents are often coupled with intravitreal foscarnet (2.4 mg/0.1 mL) and/or intravitreal ganciclovir (2 mg/0.1 mL). Inpatient management is typically reserved for patients who are unable to comply with their outpatient medication regimen or make their necessary frequent follow-up appointments.

With appropriate therapy, a reasonable outcome is possible (**Figure 38.4a**). Final visual outcome is related to the degree of macula or optic nerve involvement. Argon laser is sometimes used to track down healthy, noninvolved retina, though its utility in preventing retinal detachment (**Figure 38.4b**) is controversial. Retinal detachment is difficult to repair, typically requiring vitrectomy and silicone oil.

# Further reading

Holland GN. Standard diagnostic criteria for the acute retinal necrosis syndrome. Executive Committee of the American Uveitis Society. Am J Ophthalmol 1994; 117:663–7.

## How to approach a patient with severe vitritis

| Identify the primary pathologic clinical finding(s) | | |
|---|---|---|
| Though the view into the fundus is obscured, a discreet, white premacular lesion can be appreciated. There are clumps of vitreous cells attached in a circumferential pattern. | | |
| **Formulate a differential diagnosis** | | |
| **Most likely** | **Less likely** | **Least likely** |
| • Fungal endogenous endophthalmitis | • Bacterial endogenous endophthalmitis, toxoplasmosis, tuberculosis | • Vitreoretinal lymphoma, pars planitis, amyloidosis, syphilis, retinoblastoma |
| **Query patient history** | | |
| • Does the patient have a recent history of hospitalization?<br>• Does the patient have a history of recent fevers or night sweats?<br>• Does the patient have a history of intravenous drug use?<br>• Does the patient have a history of heart disease? | | |
| **Decide on ancillary diagnostic imaging** | | |
| Fundus photography is useful to document the extent of the process and for patient education but is not required for diagnosis. Optical coherence tomography may determine the depth of retinal infiltration, as well as demonstrate retinal edema. Fluorescein angiography may reveal vasculitis. | | |

## Ancillary diagnostic imaging interpretation

### Color photography

The media is cloudy from vitreous inflammation. Numerous white snowballs are noted in the vitreous. These are linked in a 'string of pearls' pattern. There is a discreet and circular lesion located nasal to the fovea. It appears to be 'stuck on' the retina in a preretinal location. No vascular sheathing is appreciated. The nerve is obscured, but does not appear significantly edematous (**Figure 39.1**).

### Optical coherence tomography

A diagonal cross section through the white infiltrate reveals a hyper-reflective, preretinal lesion (**Figure 39.2**). The infiltrate completely blocks light transmission (posterior shadowing) to the outer retina, retinal pigment epithelium (RPE), and choroid. The photoreceptor bands adjacent to the lesion are attenuated.

## Final diagnosis: fungal endophthalmitis, *Candida albicans*

### Epidemiology/etiology

Endophthalmitis refers to inflammation that involves both the anterior and posterior segment of the eye. It is due to infection from either an endogenous or exogenous source. Endogenous refers to the spread of organisms within the bloodstream from a more distant

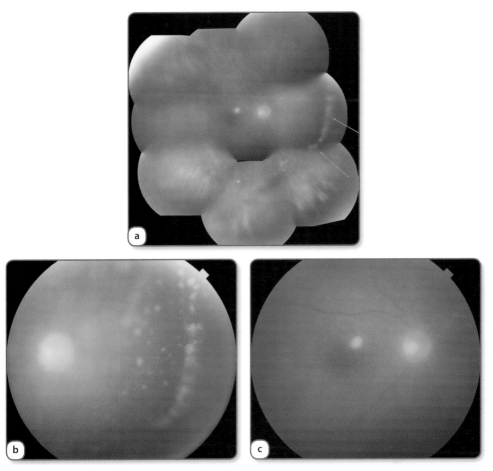

**Figure 39.1** Color photographs of the right eye are hazy due to vitreal inflammation. (a, b) A 'string of pearls' is present (red arrows). (c) There is a white preretinal lesion in the macula. The clinical findings are highly suspicious for *Candida* endophthalmitis. By courtesy of Adam Rogers, MD, Boston, MA, USA.

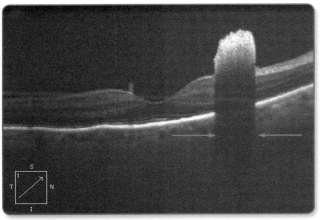

**Figure 39.2** Diagonal cross section through the infiltrate demonstrates a hyper-reflective preretinal lesion (red asterisk). There is complete posterior shadowing (red arrows). By courtesy of Adam Rogers, MD, Boston, MA, USA.

locus. Endocarditis, sepsis, indwelling catheters, and intravenous drug use are risk factors for endogenous endophthalmitis. Exogenous endophthalmitis involves direct inoculation of ocular cavities, typically from surgery or trauma. Cataract surgery and intravitreal injections are the two most common procedures associated with postoperative endophthalmitis.

The majority of cases of endophthalmitis are caused by gram-positive bacteria of the *Staphylococcus* or *Streptococcus* families. Gram-negative organisms such as *Bacillus* are more commonly seen in penetrating injuries. Fungal pathogens such as *Candida* or *Aspergillus* are the likely culprits in debilitated intensive care unit patients with presumed endogenous endophthalmitis.

## Symptoms and clinical findings

Bacterial endophthalmitis presents acutely with a red, painful, light sensitive, eye. The vision is severely affected. There can be significant eyelid swelling, conjunctival injection, and chemosis. The anterior chamber shows significant cellular reaction, often fibrinous, and a hypopyon may be present. Vitreous cell and debris can be significant, limiting the view to the posterior segment. If the view is sufficient, multifocal or confluent chorioretinitis and severe occlusive vasculitis may be noted.

Fungal endophthalmitis, on the other hand, typically has a more indolent course with days to weeks of progressive blurred vision and floaters. The main clinical findings include creamy, white, superficial, circumscribed lesions within the fundus. A significant vitritis may be seen and vitreous opacities often link to each other in a 'string of pearls' appearance.

## Treatment/prognosis/follow-up

Diagnosis is based upon gram stain and culture of aqueous and vitreous fluids. Blood cultures should be routinely ordered if there is a suspicion for an endogenous source.

The landmark Endophthalmitis-Vitrectomy Study guides treatment for the majority of cases of postsurgical endophthalmitis. Intravitreal antibiotics (+/- steroids) are injected immediately after the diagnosis is made, unless surgery is planned, and sometimes injections are repeated 48-72 hours afterwards. Newer oral agents such as moxifloxacin have been shown to achieve therapeutic levels within the posterior segment and are an attractive adjuvant to traditional therapy. Vitrectomy may be a more suitable option for those patients with fulminant disease who present with light perception vision, or for those who fail to demonstrate clinical improvement after several days of nonsurgical therapy.

If an endogenous source is found, intravenous antimicrobial therapy is warranted. Oral voriconazole may be an option for those patients with fungal endophthalmitis who prefer outpatient management and are able to be closely followed. Intravitreal pharmacotherapy is a useful adjunct to systemic treatments. Vitrectomy is typically reserved for those who do not demonstrate clinical improvement with medical therapy.

Prognosis is guarded for all types of endophthalmitis. Final outcome depends on the virulence of the offending organism, the time between symptom onset and appropriate treatment, and the extent of retinal ischemia and necrosis.

# Further reading

Breit SM, Hariprasad SM, Mieler WF, et al. Management of endogenous fungal endophthalmitis with voriconazole and caspofungin. Am J Ophthalmol 2005; 139:135–40.

Hariprasad SM, Shah GK, Mieler WF, et al. Vitreous and aqueous penetration of orally administered moxifloxacin in humans. Arch Ophthalmol 2006; 124:178–82.

Results of the Endophthalmitis Vitrectomy Study. A randomized trial of immediate vitrectomy and of intravenous antibiotics for the treatment of postoperative bacterial endopthalmitis. Endophthalmitis Vitrectomy Study Group. Arch Ophthalmol 1995; 113:1479–96.

## How to approach a patient with loss of vision and outer retinitis

| Identify the primary pathologic clinical finding(s) | | |
|---|---|---|
| There is a an area of focal chorioretinitis which is typically yellow and 'placoid-like' | | |
| **Formulate a differential diagnosis** | | |
| Most likely | Less likely | Least likely |
| • Syphilitic posterior placoid chorioretinitis | • Persistent placoid maculopathy, acute posterior multifocal placoid pigment epitheliopathy, serpiginous choroidopathy | • Intraocular tuberculosis, Vogt–Koyanagi–Harada disease, acute zonal occult outer retinopathy (AZOOR), diffuse unilateral subacute neuroretinitis, vitreoretinal lymphoma, posterior scleritis |
| **Query patient history** | | |
| • Does the patient have a recent history of viral infection, fever, weight loss or night sweats?<br>• Is the patient immunocompromised?<br>• Does the patient have any high-risk sexual practices?<br>• Does the patient have any skin rashes or genital lesions?<br>• Does the patient have a cough, shortness of breath or bloody sputum? | | |
| **Decide on ancillary diagnostic imaging** | | |
| Fundus photography is useful to document the extent of the process and and to monitor response to treatment. Optical coherence tomography may reveal outer retinal disturbances, cystoid macular edema, or subretinal fluid. Fundus autofluorescence (FAF) may demonstrate diffuse macular hyper-autofluorescence which is highly suggestive of syphilis. Fluorescein angiography may reveal optic nerve leakage, retinal vasculitis, multiple pinpoint leaks, and/or leakage into the subretinal space. | | |

## Ancillary diagnostic imaging interpretation

### Color photography

Color fundus photograph reveal blurred optic nerve head margins. There is a circular lesion involving the outer retina, retinal pigment epithelium (RPE) and choroid most evident nasal to the fovea, where there is a yellowish, crescent-shaped area of chorioretinitis (**Figure 40.1**).

### Fluorescein angiography

Fluorescein angiography may demonstrate optic nerve leakage as well as staining or leakage in areas of active retinitis (**Figure 40.2**).

## Final diagnosis: syphilitic posterior placoid chorioretinitis

### Epidemiology/etiology

Syphilis is due to infection with the spirochete *Treponema pallidum*. The primary route of transmission is through unprotected sexual contact.

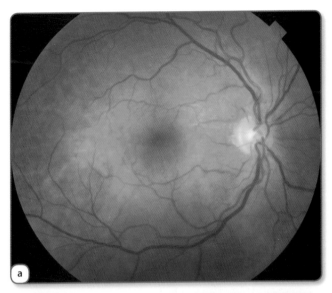

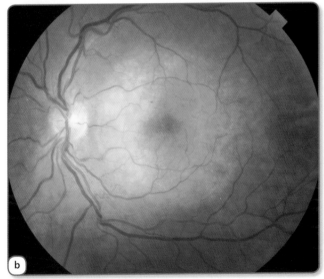

**Figure 40.1** Color photographs of the right (a) and left (b) eyes. Both optic nerves are mildly swollen. There is a placoid area of retinitis involving the left macula. By courtesy of Brian Joondeph, MD, Denver, CO, USA.

Despite programs designed to eradicate syphilis from the United States, the incidence of syphilis has actually increased over the past decade. This is due to an increase in the number of cases among men who have sex with men, a cohort of patients with high rates of HIV coinfection.

## Symptoms and clinical findings

Because of the propensity of the spirochete to invade the CNS, ocular involvement can occur at any stage of infection. Syphilis can affect almost any ocular structure and has been deemed 'the great imitator'

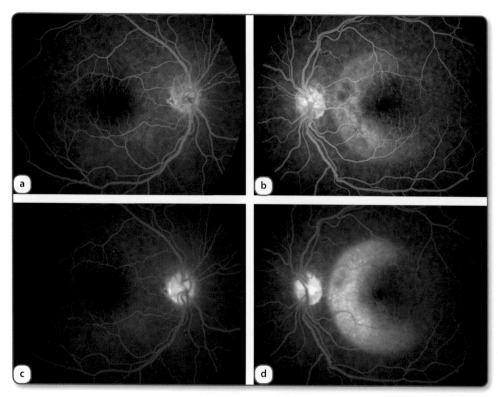

**Figure 40.2** Fluorescein angiographic images of the right (a, c) and left (b, d) eyes. Both optic nerves leak late in the study. The left eye demonstrates a crescent-shaped area of hyperfluorescence. As the study progresses, the entire lesion pools with dye. By courtesy of Brian Joondeph, MD, Denver, CO, USA.

due to the vast number of atypical presentations. It should always be on the differential of ocular inflammations.

A granulomatous uveitis with large mutton-fat keratitic precipitates should increase clinical suspicion for syphilis. Furthermore, any hypertensive (high IOP) uveitis should prompt testing for syphilis. Iris roseola, or segmental dilation of iris blood vessels, is also relatively specific for syphilis.

There are many posterior segment manifestations of syphilis, as it can affect the vitreous, retinal blood vessels, inner and outer retina, and choroid. Acute posterior placoid chorioretinitis is perhaps the most specific form of intraocular syphilis. As demonstrated in this case, it typically consists of a large, yellow, placoid lesion at the level of the RPE in the macula. Syphilis can also cause an isolated outer retinopathy, mimicking various white dot syndromes such as multiple evanescent white dot syndrome or AZOOR. It can also resemble acute retinal necrosis or other forms of peripheral retinitis. Findings felt to be specific to syphilitic retinitis include a 'ground glass' appearance and whitish-yellow focal inflammatory nodules.

## Treatment/prognosis/follow-up

Diagnosis is based upon serologic testing. Treponemal tests such as FTA-ABS and MHA-TP are highly sensitive, whereas nontreponemal tests such as RPR and VDRL are quantifiable and may be used to assess response to therapy. Lumbar puncture should be performed in patients with confirmed ocular syphilis to rule out neurologic involvement. Patients with positive testing should also be evaluated for concurrent infection with HIV, given the similar risk factors for transmission. Patients newly diagnosed with syphilis should be reported to local public health departments to facilitate partner outreach.

Infectious disease consultation is advisable. Treatment is with parenteral penicillin G for 10–14 days followed by intramuscular dosing weekly for 1 month of therapy. Topical and oral steroids may be used as an adjunct to antibiotics in patients with intraocular inflammation. Visual outcomes may be favorable if timely and aggressive therapy is administered (**Figure 40.3**).

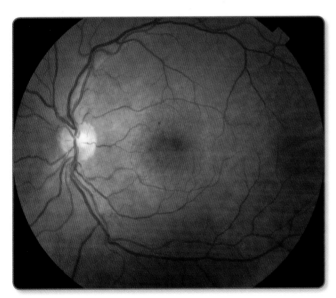

**Figure 40.3** Three months later, the chorioretinitis has resolved. Mild pigment disturbances are noted near the fovea of the left eye. By courtesy of Brian Joondeph, MD, Denver, CO, USA.

## Further reading

Chao JR, Khurana RN, Fawzi AA, et al. Syphilis: reemergence of an old adversary. Ophthalmology 2006; 113:2074–9.

Eandi CM, Neri P, Adelman RA, et al. Acute syphilitic posterior placoid chorioretinitis: report of a case series and comprehensive review of the literature. Retina 2012; 32:1915–41.

Lima BR, Mandelcorn ED, Bakshi N, et al. Syphilitic outer retinopathy. Ocul Immunol Inflamm 2014; 22(1):4–8.

## How to approach a patient with intraocular inflammation and a focal choroidal lesion

| Identify the primary pathologic clinical finding(s) | | |
|---|---|---|
| Temporal to the fovea, there is an amelanotic, irregularly shaped mass-like lesion with associated exudative detachment. | | |
| **Formulate a differential diagnosis** | | |
| Most likely | Less likely | Least likely |
| • Intraocular tuberculosis | • Endogenous endophthalmitis, amelanotic choroidal melanoma, choroidal metastases | • Posterior scleritis, sarcoidosis, toxocariasis, vitreoretinal lymphoma |
| **Query patient history** | | |
| • Where is the patient from? Any recent international travel?<br>• Does the patient have a cough, shortness of breath or bloody sputum?<br>• Does the patient have fevers, weight loss or night sweats?<br>• Is the patient immunocompromised?<br>• Does the patient use illicit drugs? | | |
| **Decide on ancillary diagnostic imaging** | | |
| Fundus photography is useful to document the extent of the process and for patient education. Furthermore, serial photography can help clinicians assess the response to treatment. Optical coherence tomography may determine the depth and extent of the lesion, as well as demonstrate retinal edema and subretinal fluid. Fluorescein angiography may reveal vasculitis, multifocal pinpoint leaks, or significant late leakage that can help to differentiate between the different diagnostic possibilities and aid in treatment decisions. | | |

## Ancillary diagnostic imaging interpretation

### Color photography

The media is cloudy, likely from vitreous inflammation. There is an irregular, whitish, subretinal or choroidal lesion with secondary exudative detachment temporal to the fovea. Radial choroidal folds can be appreciated nasal to the lesion. No vascular sheathing is appreciated (**Figure 41.1**).

### Optical coherence tomography

A vertical cross section demonstrates retinal elevation due to an irregular choroidal mass. Fibrinous subretinal fluid is noted. Deep cystic-type change can also be appreciated (**Figure 41.2**).

### Fluorescein angiography

Early frames demonstrate patchy hyperfluorescence of the mass with a few pinpoint areas of increased fluorescence. Late images show the lesion leaks extensively (**Figure 41.3**).

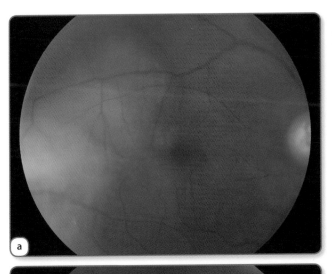

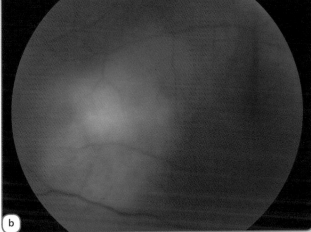

**Figure 41.1** Color photographs of the right eye: (a) macula and (b) temporal macula. There is a deep amelanotic retinal or choroidal mass temporal to the fovea. There is an associated exudative retinal detachment. By courtesy of Ying Qian, MD, Oakland, CA, USA.

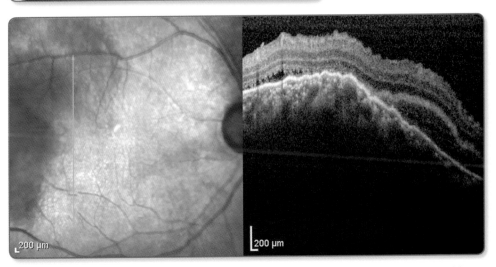

**Figure 41.2** Optical coherence tomography of the right eye, vertical slice through the lesion. There is a choroidal mass elevating the retina. There is associated subretinal fluid. By courtesy of Ying Qian, MD, Oakland, CA, USA.

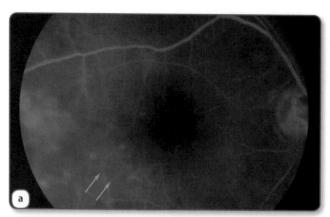

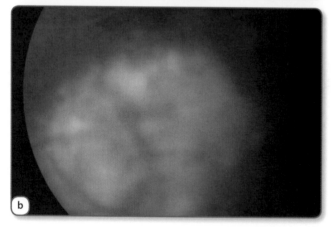

**Figure 41.3** Early (a) angiographic image centered on the fovea reveals areas of pinpoint and diffuse leakage temporal to the fovea. Choroidal folds are nicely illustrated (blue arrows). (b) As the study progresses, the lesion leaks extensively. By courtesy of Ying Qian, MD, Oakland, CA, USA.

# Final diagnosis: intraocular tuberculosis

## Epidemiology/etiology

Intraocular tuberculosis is a relatively rare cause of posterior uveitis in the United States, but is much higher worldwide especially in Southeast Asia and parts of Africa. The majority of cases in the US involve either foreign-born patients or immunocompromised patients, especially those with HIV.

*Mycobacterium tuberculosis* is an acid-fast bacillus that is responsible for the multisystem clinical manifestations of tuberculosis. Infection spreads by airborne transmission. As such, the lungs are the most commonly affected organs. Hematogenous spread of the organism can lead to extrapulmonary involvement. Intraocular involvement can occur in patients with or without concurrent pulmonary or systemic disease.

## Symptoms and clinical findings

TB can involve all parts of the eye. A granulomatous anterior uveitis with large, mutton fat keratitic precipitates is commonly seen. A significant vitritis with snowballs can also be found.

Posterior uveitis is the most common manifestation of intraocular TB. Choroidal tubercles are deep, yellow, elevated lesions found most often in the posterior pole. They may be unilateral or bilateral. These may grow into tuberculomas, which are large tumor-like lesions that can be associated with exudative retinal detachment. These tumors can rupture through Bruch's membrane and lead to severe panophthalmitis.

Retinal vasculitis due to TB can be severe and may lead to peripheral nonperfusion with secondary neovascularization and vitreous hemorrhage. In fact, there is speculation that many cases of Eales' disease are due to undiagnosed infection with *Mycobacterium tuberculosis*. Veins are typically more affected than arteries and Kyrieleis plaques can be seen in the walls of arterioles following the acute inflammatory phase.

TB can also cause a serpiginous-like choroidopathy, a variant which is commonly seen in India. Two patterns may be seen: (1) multifocal inflammatory choroidal lesions that ultimately coalesce, resembling ampiginous choroidopathy and (2) Solitary macular placoid lesion that grows in a pseuopod fashion, resembling persistent placoid maculopathy.

## Treatment/prognosis/follow-up

Diagnosis is made based upon risk factors, clinical appearance, imaging results, cultures, PCR, and laboratory testing. Treatment should be instituted under the guidance of an infectious disease specialist. Ocular TB is initially treated in a manner similar to pulmonary TB with four-drug pharmacotherapy consisting of INH, rifampin, pyrazinamide, and ethambutol.

Prognosis may be good if appropriate and aggressive treatment is instituted in a timely fashion (**Figure 41.4**). Topical, periocular, oral, and intravitreal steroids may be used as an adjuvant to treat significant ocular inflammation. Patients also must be monitored closely for any medication-related side effects. For instance, ethambutol and INH have been linked to optic neuropathy.

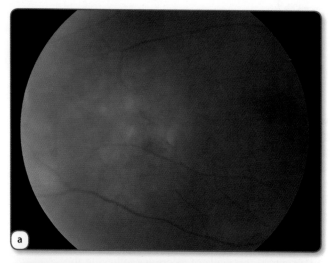

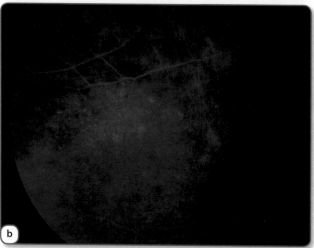

**Figure 41.4** Color photograph (a) and late angiographic image (b) of the right eye after 4 weeks of medical treatment. The lesion has regressed. There is some moderate RPE mottling and atrophy. No associated subretinal fluid is present and the choroidal folds have resolved. Five minutes after dye infusion, the lesion is nearly silent angiographically with only a few points of hyperfluorescence remaining. By courtesy of Ying Qian, MD, Oakland, CA, USA.

## Further reading

Yeh S, Sen HN, Colyer M, et al. Update on ocular tuberculosis. Curr Opin Ophthalmol 2012; 23:551–6.
Zhang M, Zhang J, Liu Y. Clinical presentations and therapeutic effect of presumed choroidal tuberculosis. Retina 2012; 32:805–13.

# Unilateral acute idiopathic maculopathy

## How to approach a patient with acute loss of vision, recent flu-like illness, and a subretinal lesion

| Identify the primary pathologic clinical finding(s) | | |
|---|---|---|
| Inferior to the fovea there is a yellowish, oval-shaped, subretinal or choroidal lesion. | | |
| **Formulate a differential diagnosis** | | |
| Most likely | Less likely | Least likely |
| • Unilateral acute idiopathic maculopathy (UAIM) | • Fibrinous central serous retinopathy, idiopathic CNV, infectious focal choroiditis, sarcoidosis, acute posterior multifocal placoid pigment epitheliopathy (APMPPE) | • Choroidal hemangioma, choroidal metastases, amelanotic nevus, vitreoretinal lymphoma |
| **Query patient history** | | |
| • Does the patient have a history of recent fever, flu, sore throat or laryngitis? <br> • Does the patient have any new rashes particularly on the hands or feet? <br> • Does the patient have any cough, shortness of breath or bloody sputum? <br> • Is the patient pregnant? <br> • Has the patient been experiencing a recent increase in stress? <br> • Is the patient myopic? <br> • Does the patient have a history of cancer? | | |
| **Decide on ancillary diagnostic imaging** | | |
| Fundus photography is useful to document the extent of the process and for patient education. Furthermore, serial photography can help clinicians assess the response to treatment. Optical coherence tomography (OCT) may determine the depth and extent of the lesion, as well as demonstrate retinal edema and subretinal fluid. Fluorescein angiography (FA) is essential in differentiating between the different diagnostic possibilities. ICG is the best imaging modality to identify choroidal hemangioma, if still considered a possible etiology after OCT testing. | | |

## Ancillary diagnostic imaging interpretation

### Color photography

There is a yellowish, deep oval-shaped lesion inferior to the fovea, which is amorphous with indistinct borders. There does not appear to be a gutter of subretinal fluid. No other retinal pigment epithelial changes are noted elsewhere in either macula. There is no hemorrhage or signs of myopic degeneration (**Figure 42.1**).

### Optical coherence tomography

Time-domain OCT reveals an area of thickening inferotemporal to the fovea. A vertical slice through the lesion demonstrates subtle outer retinal and RPE abnormalities. No intraretinal or subretinal fluid is noted.

One month after presentation, spectral-domain OCT was

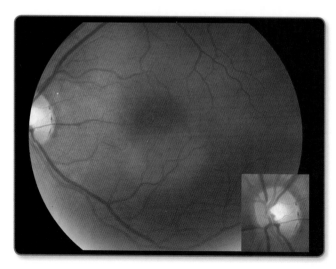

**Figure 42.1** Color photograph of the left eye demonstrates an oval-shaped subretinal/choroidal lesion inferior to the fovea. There is no associated hemorrhage or subretinal fluid.

performed. A vertical cross section through the lesion demonstrates it to be irregular and isoreflective. It resides in a subretinal location. The RPE appears to be involved as well. Overlying the lesion, the outer retinal bands are lost. There is no subretinal fluid or intraretinal fluid. The choroid underlying the lesion appears thickened (**Figure 42.2**).

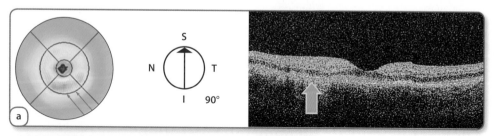

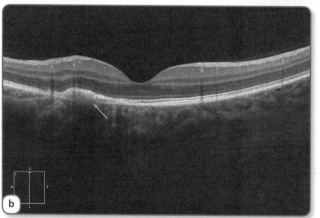

**Figure 42.2** Time domain (a) optical coherence tomography (OCT) of the left eye at presentation. The color map (red arrows) reveals irregular thickening inferotemporal to the fovea. A vertical section demonstrates abnormalities of the outer retina and RPE (thick blue arrow). Spectral domain (b) OCT, vertical cross section, performed 1 month after presentation. The lesion (blue arrow) involves the space between the external limiting membrane and Bruch's membrane. The photoreceptors and the RPE are involved. The inner-segment/outer-segment (IS/OS) ellipsoid and OS-RPE lines are absent.

## Fluorescein angiography

Early frames demonstrate patchy hyperfluorescence of the lesion. As the study progresses, the lesion completely fills and stains with dye, with relatively increased hyperfluorescence and leakage at the superior border. The margins of the lesion are wedge-shaped (**Figure 42.3**).

# Final diagnosis: UAIM

## Epidemiology/etiology

Originally described by Yannuzzi in 1991, UAIM is an uncommon disorder typically affecting young or middle-aged adults. It has been linked to Coxsackievirus and hand-foot-mouth disease. There may be seasonality to its presentation (late summer) that gives additional credence to the relationship with Coxsackievirus. Inflammation of the outer retina, RPE and/or choroid likely produces the characteristic appearance.

## Symptoms and clinical findings

Patients typically present with acute-onset, unilateral, painless vision loss days or weeks after a flu-like illness. There usually is a central or paracentral scotoma in the involved eye.

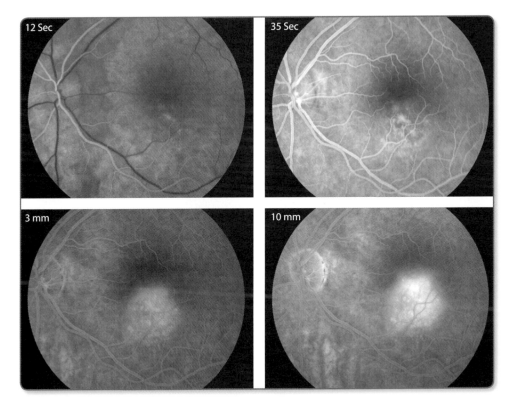

**Figure 42.3** Angiographic images of the left eye at presentation. There is early spotty hyperfluorescence with complete late staining of the lesion and leakage at the superior border.

Classic findings consist of an intermediate-sized, solitary, yellowish-gray, placoid lesion at the level of the RPE, which may be associated with adjacent intraretinal hemorrhages. Papillitis, mild vitreous inflammation, and bilateral presentations have been described as well.

The results of multimodality imaging are critical in differentiating UAIM from other potential diagnoses. The location of the lesion on OCT in a subretinal location rules out choroidal disorders and tumors. The leakage pattern on FA is atypical for CSCR, Harada's disease or APMPPE. Myopic or idiopathic CNV is another consideration, but a yellowish subretinal lesion would be atypical for neovascular tissue.

## Treatment/prognosis/follow-up

The majority of patients recover their vision entirely without treatment. over weeks to months. Because it remains unknown if UAIM is directly due to an infectious agent or indirectly from an aberrant immune response, treatment with steroids is controversial.

Complications of UAIM include choroidal neovascularization and development of a 'bull's-eye' pattern of macular atrophy.

## Further reading

Freund KB, Yannuzzi LA, Barile GR, et al. The expanding clinical spectrum of unilateral acute idiopathic maculopathy. Arch Ophthalmol 1996; 114:555–9.

# 47

# Acute macular neuroretinopathy

## How to approach a patient with new visual symptoms and the appearance of perifoveal spots

| Identify the primary pathologic clinical finding(s) | | |
|---|---|---|
| The color photos and red-free images reveal petaloid lesions just superior to the fovea in both eyes. | | |
| **Formulate a differential diagnosis** | | |
| Most likely | Less likely | Least likely |
| • Acute macular neuroretinopathy (AMNR) | • Acute retinal pigment epithelitis, solar maculopathy, Welder's maculopathy | • Multiple evanescent white dot syndrome, 'Poppers' maculopathy |
| **Query patient history** | | |
| • Has the patient been sick recently?<br>• Has the patient been taking any medications?<br>• Has the patient been drinking a lot of caffeine?<br>• Has the patient had recent surgery? Was there significant<br>• blood loss?<br>• Has the patient had significant changes in blood pressure? | | |
| **Decide on ancillary diagnostic imaging** | | |
| Fundus photography may be useful to document the extent of the lesions and for patient education. Red-free pictures, near-infrared photos, and optical coherence tomography (OCT) fundus images often more readily show the macular abnormalities. OCT can also demonstrate hyper-reflective bands in the middle or outer retina. As the disease evolves, it can also reveal additional outer retinal abnormalities such as thinning of the nuclear and plexiform layers and loss and disruption of the outer retina. Fluorescein angiography and indocyanine green angiography (ICGA) help to rule out other possible causes of vision loss. | | |

## Ancillary diagnostic imaging interpretation

### Color photography

Color photography reveals subtle wedge-shaped reddish-brown lesions just superior to the fovea in each eye (**Figure 47.1a**). The optic nerves and vasculature appear within normal limits.

### Red-free imaging

Red-free imaging highlights the lesions more clearly (**Figure 47.1b**). The lesions appear to involve the fovea.

### Optical coherence tomography

In the right eye, there is a hyper-reflective band in the region of the outer nuclear layer within the fovea. It involves the outer retinal bands as well. The retinal pigment epithelium (RPE) appears unaffected. Nasal to this there is an additional area of outer retinal disruption and outer nuclear layer involvement. A middle limiting membrane can be

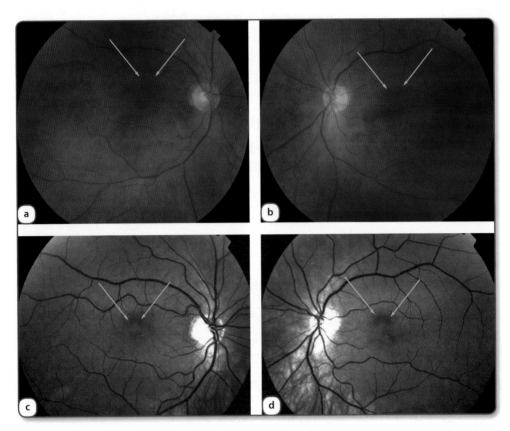

**Figure 47.1** Color photographs (a,b) and red-free images (c,d) of the right and left eye. The brightness of the color photo was increased by 30% to better demonstrate the abnormalities. Blue arrows point to subtle petaloid lesions just above the fovea in each eye. The lesions are much better seen using red-free (red arrows) photography.

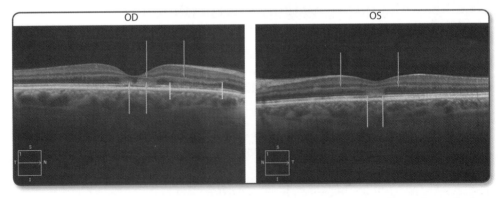

**Figure 47.2** Optical coherence tomographic images. Blue arrows illustrate hyper-reflective lesions that involve the outer nuclear layer and the photoreceptor bands in both eyes. There is an area of central clearing in the right eye. The RPE appears intact. The yellow arrows bracket another wedge-shaped area of retinal involvement in the right eye. Middle limiting membranes can be appreciated (red arrows).

appreciated (**Figure 47.2a**).

In the left eye, there is a hyper-reflective band in the foveal region. It reaches from the outer plexiform layer to the anterior aspect of the RPE. A middle limiting membrane again is noted (**Figure 47.2b**).

## Indocyanine green angiography

Mid-phase ICGA of both eyes is within normal limits (**Figure 47.3**).

# Final diagnosis: acute macular neuroretinopathy

## Epidemiology/etiology

AMNR typically affects females aged 20–50 years. Though the cause of this disorder is unknown, risk factors such as systemic hypotension and concomitant use of sympathomimetics like caffeine or epinephrine

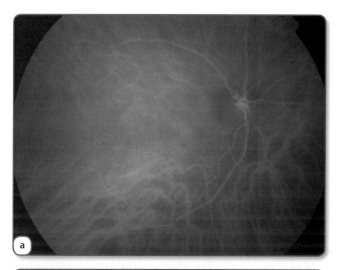

**Figure 47.3** Mid-phase indocyanine green angiographic images of the right (a) and left (b) eyes are within normal limits.

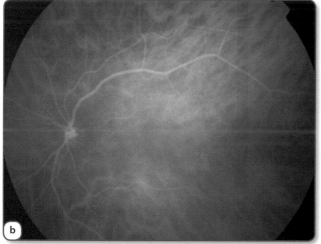

suggest an ischemic etiology. Visual symptoms due to acute macular neuroretinopathy (AMNR) can also be preceded by a flu-like illness, which raises the possibility of an infectious or autoimmune cause for this disorder.

## Symptoms and clinical findings

Patients typically experience sudden blurred vision in one or both eyes. They may complain of one or multiple paracentral scotomas.

Anterior segment or vitreous inflammation is typically absent. The characteristic findings consist of multiple reddish-brown wedge-shaped or clover-leaf lesions surrounding and pointing toward the fovea. The lesions can be very subtle to observe with direct illumination. They are much better exposed with red-free and near-infrared photography.

OCT is invaluable in the diagnosis of AMNR. A C-scan or OCT fundus image often is the best imaging modality to identify subtle retinal lesions. Cross-sectional retinal slices may reveal outer retinal lesions involving the outer nuclear layer and photoreceptor bands, as seen in this case. These lesions may be the result of ischemia to the deep capillary plexus, located at the outermost portion of the inner nuclear layer. The appearance of a tomographic middle limiting membrane in some of these patients provides more evidence in support of an ischemic etiology.

## Treatment/prognosis/follow-up

There is no evidence that any treatment alters the outcome of these patients. Many patients will be left with residual scotoma. Severe permanent central vision loss is rare.

## Further reading

Fawzi AA, Pappuru RR, Sarraf D, et al. Acute macular neuroretinopathy: long-term insights revealed by multimodal imaging. Retina 2012; 32:1500–1513.

Sarraf D, Rahimy E, Fawzi AA, et al. Paracentral acute middle maculopathy: a new variant of acute macular neuroretinopathy associated with retinal capillary ischemia. JAMA Ophthalmol 2013; 131:1275–87.

# 48

# Punctate inner choroidopathy

## How to approach a patient with visual symptoms and punched-out lesions in the retina

| Identify the primary pathologic clinical finding(s) | | |
|---|---|---|
| Both eyes show numerous punched-out lesions scattered throughout the macula and nasal periphery. Some of the lesions are pigmented. There is a grey-green membrane just inferior to the fovea of the right eye. | | |

| Formulate a differential diagnosis | | |
|---|---|---|
| **Most likely** | **Less likely** | **Least likely** |
| • Punctate inner choroidopathy (PIC) | • Multifocal choroiditis, presumed ocular histoplasmosis syndrome (POHS), West Nile chorioretinopathy | • Sarcoid-related choroiditis, coccidioidomycosis, vitreoretinal lymphoma, birdshot choroidopathy, myopic degeneration |

| Query patient history |
|---|
| • Has the patient been sick lately? Any fevers?<br>• Is the patient immunocompromised?<br>• Does the patient work with animals?<br>• Any exposure to bats or birds?<br>• Is the patient myopic?<br>• Does the patient have shortness of breath? |

| Decide on ancillary diagnostic imaging |
|---|
| Fundus photography is useful to document the extent of the abnormalities and for patient education. Red-free photos can also help to highlight the lesions. Optical coherence tomography can aid in the identification of secondary choroidal neovascular (CNV) membranes. Fluorescein angiography (FA) is helpful in differentiating this condition from other possibilities and for detecting the presence of CNV. Indocyanine green angiography may demonstrate subclinical lesions, aiding in the diagnosis of unusual cases. As the disease progresses, FAF is helpful in assessing the state of the retinal pigment epithelium. |

## Ancillary diagnostic imaging interpretation

### Color photography

Color photography demonstrates multiple punched-out lesions with varying degrees of pigmentation scattered in the macula and around the optic nerve. Optic nerve edema, peripapillary scarring and vitritis are absent. No circumferential lesions are noted in the periphery. Just inferior to the fovea in the right eye is a grey-green membrane, without associated hemorrhage (**Figure 48.1**).

### Optical coherence tomography

Thickness map of the right eye reveals an area of thickening just inferior to the fovea. Serial horizontal cross sections demonstrate a subretinal lesion concerning for choroidal neovascularization. An area of outer retina and retinal pigment epithelium (RPE) atrophy is also noted (**Figure 48.2**).

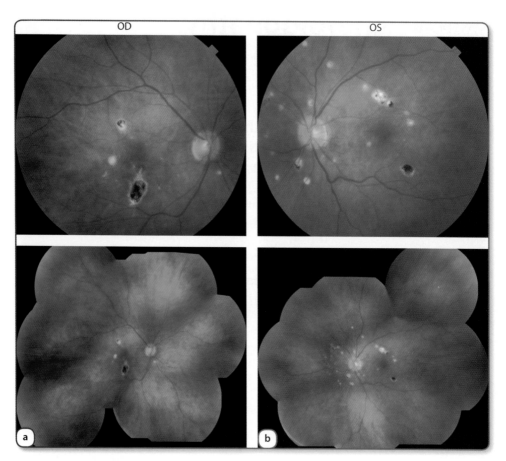

**Figure 48.1** Color photographs of the right (a) and left (b) eyes demonstrate multiple punched-out lesions scattered in the macula and around the optic nerve. Some are pigmented. There is a grey-green membrane adjacent to a pigmented scar inferior to the fovea in the right eye. Of note, there are no peripapillary changes.

## Red-free imaging

Red-free imaging highlights the lesions clearly (**Figure 48.3a**).

## Fluorescein angiography

FA confirms the presence of CNV as demonstrated by a progressive juxtafoveal leak at the superior edge of a large pigmented punched-out lesion (**Figure 48.3b**).

## Final diagnosis: punctate inner choroidopathy

## Epidemiology/etiology

Punctate inner choroidopathy (PIC) typically affects myopic females aged 20–40 years. The etiology is unknown. Current research points to an altered immune response to a still unidentified infectious antigen.

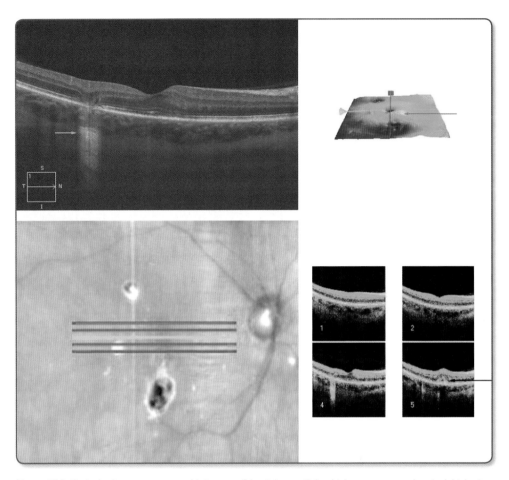

**Figure 48.2** Optical coherence tomographic images of the right eye. Color thickness map reveals retinal thickening inferior to the fovea (red arrow). Serial horizontal B scans through the fovea reveal a subretinal lesion concerning for choroidal neovascularization (black arrow). A section through an atrophic lesion demonstrates loss of the outer nuclear and outer retinal and RPE bands with increased light penetration to the choroid (blue arrow).

## Symptoms and clinical findings

Patients typically present with blurred vision, metamorphopsia, photopsias, and/or paracentral scotomas.

By definition, there is an absence of anterior or posterior segment inflammation. At the onset of the disease, the characteristic findings consist of multiple white-yellow chorioretinal infiltrates scattered throughout the macula. The lesions may extend around the optic nerve and out to the mid-periphery. The lesions are bilateral in the majority of cases. As time passes, these lesions evolve into punched-out atrophic scars, many with a pigmented border.

The lack of intraocular inflammation rules out multifocal choroiditis. Patients with presumed ocular histoplasmosis (POHS) are from endemic areas and typically display peripapillary atrophy

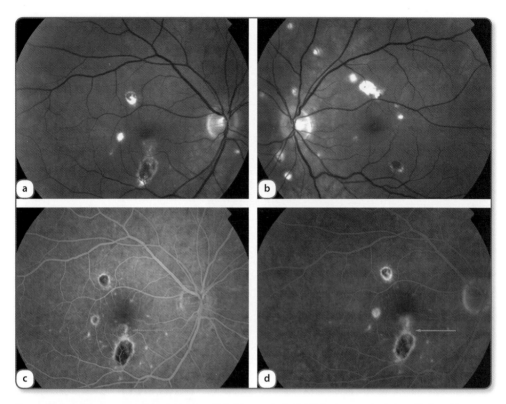

**Figure 48.3** Red-free images of the right (a) and left (b) eyes nicely highlight the macular lesions. Early and late angiographic images of the right eye (c, d) reveal an area of increasing fluorescence inferior to the fovea, consistent with choroidal neovascularization (red arrows).

or pigmentation. The peripheral atrophic lesions in POHS may also form a linear or circumferential pattern, another feature that helps to differentiate it from PIC.

## Treatment/prognosis/follow-up

PIC is typically a self-limiting disease and can often be managed conservatively with excellent visual prognosis. However, patients with foveal-threatening lesions may benefit from systemic, periocular or intravitreal steroids in hopes of arresting the disease process. The most common cause of vision loss is choroidal neovascularization, which occurs in 40–75% of patients. Secondary CNV is typically managed with anti-VEGF agents solely or in combination with local steroid therapy.

The prognosis for PIC without CNV is favorable, with the vast majority of eyes maintaining vision >20/25. Patients with CNV have a worse prognosis. Twenty percent of those eyes will have vision worse than 20/200.

## Further reading

Brown J Jr, Folk JC, Reddy CV, et al. Visual prognosis of multifocal choroiditis, punctate inner choroidopathy, and the diffuse subretinal fibrosis syndrome. Ophthalmology 1996; 103:1100–105.
Patel KH, Birnbaum AD, Tessler HH, Goldstein DA. Presentation and outcome of patients with punctate inner choroidopathy at a tertiary referral center. Retina 2011; 31:1387–91.

# 49

# Birdshot chorioretinopathy

## How to approach a patient with new visual symptoms and multiple new yellow lesions in the retina

| Identify the primary pathologic clinical finding(s) | | |
|---|---|---|
| In each eye, there are yellow, circular, creamy lesions that radiate from the optic nerve to the periphery. The lesions are also scattered around the fovea. They appear to reside either in the retinal pigment epithelium (RPE) or choroid. | | |
| **Formulate a differential diagnosis** | | |
| **Most likely** | **Less likely** | **Least likely** |
| • Birdshot chorioretinopathy | • Sarcoid choroiditis, multifocal choroiditis, benign reactive lymphoid hyperplasia | • Vitreoretinal lymphoma |
| **Query patient history** | | |
| • Is the patient seeing floaters or flashes?<br>• Are there symptoms in one or both eyes?<br>• Any difficulty with night vision?<br>• Any shortness of breath on limited exertion? | | |
| **Decide on ancillary diagnostic imaging** | | |
| Fundus photography is useful to document the extent of the lesions and for patient education. Red-free photographs can also help to highlight the lesions. Indocyanine green angiography (ICGA) often reveals the disease to be more widespread than is readily appreciated clinically. Optical coherence tomography (OCT) can demonstrate the presence of macular edema. Fluorescein angiography is not as helpful in differentiating these conditions – CME can be detected readily by OCT and other angiographic findings are not specific to any one diagnosis. As the disease progresses, FAF is helpful in assessing the state of the retinal pigment epithelium. | | |

## Ancillary diagnostic imaging interpretation

### Color photography

Color photography demonstrates numerous circular, creamy lesions at the level of the RPE or choroid (**Figure 49.1**). They appear to radiate out from the optic nerve and are scattered symmetrically across the fundus. Some lesions follow the choroid vasculature (choroidotropic).

### Red-free imaging

Red-free imaging highlights the lesions clearly (**Figure 49.2**). Mild cellophane change is noted bilaterally.

### Indocyanine green angiography

Late-phase ICGA reveals numerous hypofluorescent lesions. Many more lesions are evident than can be appreciated clinically (**Figure 49.3**).

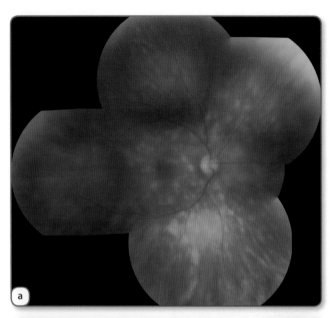

**Figure 49.1** Color montage photographs of the right (a) and left (b) eyes. In both eyes, there are numerous yellow-orange lesions radiating out from the optic nerve to the periphery. They seem to follow the choroidal vasculature. In the macula, the lesions encircle the fovea.

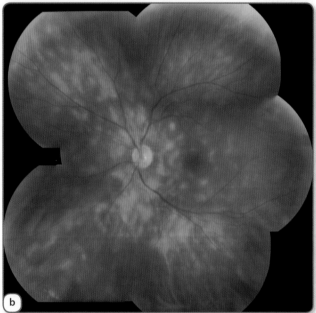

# Final diagnosis: birdshot chorioretinopathy

## Epidemiology/etiology

Birdshot chorioretinopathy affects middle-aged adults, with an average age at diagnosis of 50 years. There is no clear gender predilection, though some studies have demonstrated a slight female preference.

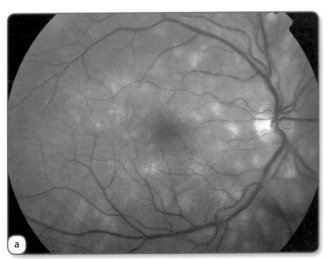

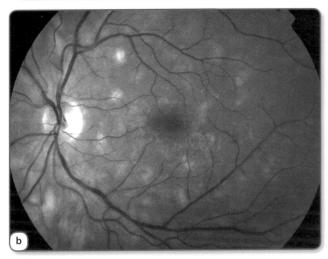

**Figure 49.2** Red-free photography of the right (a) and left (b) eyes highlights the lesions. They are concentrated in the peripapillary locations and surround the fovea in each eye. There is a mild epiretinal membrane in the left eye.

Though the cause is unknown, there is a strong relationship (>90%) with the HLA-A29 haplotype.

## Symptoms and clinical findings

Acutely, patients experience blurred vision in one or both eyes. They complain of floaters and peripheral photopsias. Other presenting symptoms may include night vision difficulties and poor color discrimination.

Visual acuity is only mildly affected at presentation, usually in the 20/60 range. There is typically very little anterior segment inflammation. Anterior vitreous cells are invariably present, but the presence of snowballs or snowbanks would be unusual for birdshot. The nerve can be mildly edematous and foveal cystic changes or epiretinal membrane may be present. Characteristic findings consist

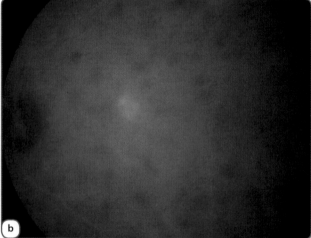

**Figure 49.3** Late indocyanine green angiographic (ICGA) images of the right (a) and left (b) eyes. The lesions of birdshot are hypofluorescent, either from blocking or choroidal ischemia. More lesions are detected by ICGA than can be appreciated clinically.

of multiple, flat, cream-colored lesions that appear to radiate out from the optic nerve. Acute lesions appear creamy and indistinct. As time evolves, these lesions are noted to be more punched-out and discrete without significant pigmentation.

Laboratory evaluation for HLA-A29 is indicated and helps solidify the diagnosis.

## Treatment/prognosis/follow-up

Like other autoimmune disease, birdshot is chronic and recurrent. At presentation, systemic steroids are used to control the inflammation. Immunomodulatory therapy, typically cyclosporine, is the mainstay of chronic treatment, given the significant morbidity of long-term systemic steroid therapy. Intraocular steroids may be used as an adjuvant to decrease the intensity of systemic therapy and/or treat local complications of the disease.

The most common cause of vision loss in birdshot is cystoid macula edema. Macular and peripapillary CNV is not uncommon. For many patients, prompt and aggressive therapy can preserve visual acuity and prevent many of the blinding complications of the disease. However, a significant minority of patients will ultimately develop permanent vision loss and nyctalopia from either optic atrophy or diffuse retinal atrophy.

## Further reading

Shah KH, Levinson RD, Yu F, et al. Birdshot chorioretinopathy. Surv Ophthalmol 2005; 50:519–41.

# 50

# Intermediate uveitis

## How to approach a patient with floaters, decreased vision, and vitreous inflammation

| Identify the primary pathologic clinical finding(s) | | |
| --- | --- | --- |
| Both eyes demonstrate a hazy view of the posterior pole with loss of the foveal light reflex. | | |
| **Formulate a differential diagnosis** | | |
| Most likely | Less likely | Least likely |
| • Intermediate uveitis (pars planitis) | • Multiple sclerosis, sarcoidosis, syphilis, Lyme disease, ocular tuberculosis | • Vitreomacular traction, epiretinal membrane |
| **Query patient history** | | |
| • Does the patient have any medical problems? Any shortness of breath?<br>• Any weakness, numbness or tingling?<br>• Is the patient sexually active? Any history of sexually transmitted diseases?<br>• Any history of new skin rashes? Any genital sores or rashes?<br>• Any tick bites? | | |
| **Decide on ancillary diagnostic imaging** | | |
| Fundus photography is useful to document vitritis, optic nerve swelling, or retinal phlebitis. Optical coherence tomography (OCT) of the macula can demonstrate cystoid macular edema. Widefield fluorescein angiography (FA) may reveal peripheral venous leakage and cystoid macular edema. | | |

## Ancillary diagnostic imaging interpretation

### Color photography

Color fundus photographs show loss of the foveal light reflex and a mildly hazy view due to vitritis (**Figure 50.1**). Neither optic disc swelling nor retinal phlebitis is present.

### Optical coherence tomography

OCT of each eye reveals cystoid macular edema, left worse than right. The swelling involves the inner nuclear layer and Henle's layer. In both eyes, there is a small amount of subfoveal fluid (**Figure 50.2a**).

Treatment of each eye with a posterior sub-Tenon's triamcinolone injection led to the resolution of macular edema (**Figure 50.2b**).

### Fluorescein angiography

The early frames are unremarkable. Late frames show a late petaloid leak in both eyes (**Figure 50.3**). The nerves also demonstrate mild late hyperfluorescence. There is no evidence of vasculitis in these images.

## Final diagnosis: intermediate uveitis

### Epidemiology/etiology

Pars planitis typically affects children and young adults with peaks occurring between the ages of 5–15 years and 25–35 years.

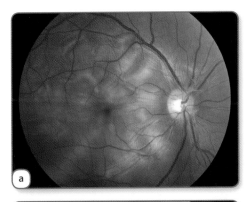
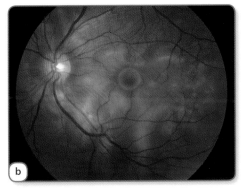
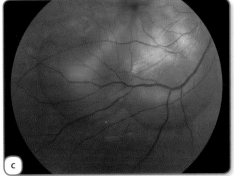

**Figure 51.1** Color fundus photographs of the right and left macula (a, b) and an area inferior to the macula of the right eye (c). There are multiple serous detachments in each eye. There appears to be deep yellow infiltrates underlying these exudative detachments. The subretinal fluid in the right eye gravitates inferiorly creating two 'tear-drop' detachments. In the left eye, there is also a pocket of subfoveal fluid that is encircled by a yellow ring.

in both eyes (**Figure 51.3a**). As the study progresses, these dots and areas progressively become more hyperfluorescent as dye pools into the subretinal space (**Figure 51.3b**).

# Final diagnosis: VKH syndrome

## Epidemiology/etiology

VKH mostly affects people of dark pigmentation. As such, it is more common in patients from Asian, Middle Eastern, Native American, and Hispanic descent. There is a female predominance.

An autoimmune process directed against melanocytes is thought be responsible for the characteristic clinical features. There is an association with HLA-DR4, which further suggests an aberrant immune response to either an infectious or local antigen.

## Symptoms and clinical findings

VKH is a multisystemic inflammatory condition with dermatologic, neurologic, and ophthalmic involvement. Patients most frequently present after a flu-like illness with symptoms such as malaise, headache, and meningismus (with associated CSF pleocytosis). This is called the prodromal phase. During this stage, sensitivity to touch of the hair and

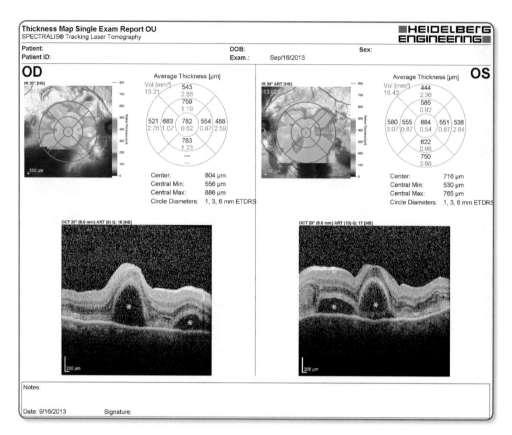

**Figure 51.2** Optical coherence tomography reveals multiple pockets of subretinal fluid in both eyes (asterisks). There is fibrin or other infiltrative/inflammatory material filling the subretinal space as well (blue asterisks). Because enhanced-depth imaging was not performed, the thickness of the choroid cannot be reliably measured.

skin can also be noted. Inner ear disorders, such as tinnitus and vertigo, and high-frequency hearing loss can also develop during this phase. Cranial nerve palsies are rarely seen.

Visual symptoms such as photophobia, eye pain, decreased vision, and distortion ultimately develop. This is the uveitic phase, which may last for 2–6 weeks. Examination shows severe bilateral granulomatous uveitis with mild vitritis, yellow-white retinal exudates in the retinal pigment epithelium and serous retinal detachment. Dalen-Fuchs nodules may be apparent. Optic disc edema is a frequent finding.

After resolution of the acute uveitis, patients enter the convalescent phase characterized by depigmented areas at the limbus, called Sugiura's sign. The retina develops a characteristic 'sunset glow' appearance, as the newly depigmented choroid takes on a red-orange hue. Furthermore, poliosis of the scalp, eyebrow, eyelashes, and vitiligo of periocular and facial skin may occur.

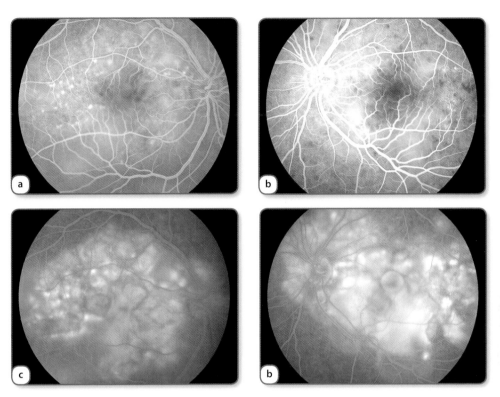

**Figure 51.3** Fluorescein angiography, early (a) and late (b) images. There is diffuse early hyperfluorescence OU and areas of pinpoint hyperfluorescence temporally OU. As the study progresses, there is extensive pooling of dye into the subretinal space and numerous areas of leakage.

## Treatment/prognosis/follow-up

VKH is very responsive to systemic corticosteroids. Steroid-sparing immunomodulatory therapies are often added to reduce the likelihood of disease recurrence and to minimize steroid-induced side effects. Visual prognosis can be reasonable with prompt and aggressive treatment. Despite this, long-term sequelae such as angle closure or steroid-induced glaucoma, pigment epithelial hyperplasia or atrophy, subretinal fibrosis and choroidal neovascularization may lead to permanent vision loss.

# Further reading

Damico FM, Kiss S, Young LH. Vogt-Koyanagi-Harada disease. Semin Ophthalmol 2005; 20:183–90.

# How to approach a patient with intraocular inflammation and retinal vasculitis

| Identify the primary pathologic clinical finding(s) | | |
|---|---|---|
| The montage photograph demonstrates sheathing of the veins within the inferior and inferior-nasal quadrants. There are numerous intraretinal hemorrhages in the periphery, some with white centers. | | |
| **Formulate a differential diagnosis** | | |
| **Most likely** | **Less likely** | **Least likely** |
| • Behçet's disease | • Sarcoidosis, systemic lupus erythematosus, polyarteritis nodosa, Eales' disease, idiopathic frosted-branch angiitis, cat scratch disease | • Cytomegalovirus retinitis, syphilis, acute retinal necrosis, leukemia, multiple sclerosis |
| **Query patient history** | | |
| • Does the patient have any oral and/or genital ulcers?<br>• What is the patient's ethnic background? Any international travel?<br>• Any skin rashes?<br>• Does the patient have any immune deficieny or HIV? | | |
| **Decide on ancillary diagnostic imaging** | | |
| Fundus photography is useful to document the extent of the abnormalities and for patient education. Optical coherence tomography can demonstrate macular edema and areas of inner retinal thickening and hyperreflectivity, findings suggestive of an ischemic or occlusive process. Fluorescein angiography (FA) is essential to evaluate for retinal vasculitis and to assess the degree of retinal ischemia. FA also reveals the distribution of the vasculitis: arterial, venous, or both (**Table 52.1**). | | |

# Ancillary diagnostic imaging interpretation

## Color photography

Fundus photograph of the left eye demonstrates sheathing of the veins coursing inferiorly from the optic nerve, which is hyperemic. An inflammatory exudation encases the affected vessels, causing the involved area to resemble a 'frosted branch.' Intraretinal hemorrhages track the course of the vessels. Numerous circular hemorrhages are also noted in the far periphery, some with white centers (**Figure 52.1**).

## Fluorescein angiography

Early frames focused on the inferior retina show sluggish filling of inferior arteries. There is a 'leading edge' of dye inflow. An occluded 'ghost' artery is noted. Vascular pruning and early downstream anastomoses can be seen in this area. As the study progresses, the inflamed vessels leak extensively (**Figures 52.2** and **52.3**).

| Table 52.1 Differential diagnosis of retinal vasculitis | |
| --- | --- |
| **Vessels involved** | **Differential diagnosis** |
| Veins (phlebitis) | Behçet's disease, tuberculosis, sarcoidosis, multiple sclerosis, pars planitis, Eales' disease, frosted branch angiitis*, birdshot retinochoroidopathy, acute multifocal hemorrhagic retinal vasculitis, human immunodeficiency virus, human T-cell lymphoma virus, cytomegalovirus, Lyme disease*, lymphoma* |
| Arteries (arteritis) | Acute retinal necrosis, progressive outer retinal necrosis (varicella zoster virus), idiopathic retinal vasculitis, aneurysms and neuroretinitis (IRVAN), systemic lupus erythematosus (SLE), polyarteritis nodosa (PAN), granulomatosis with polyangiitis*, Churg–Strauss syndrome, cryoglobulinemia, Susac's syndrome, syphilis*, herpes simplex virus, Epstein–Barr virus, toxoplasmosis*, cat scratch disease*, Crohn's disease*, relapsing polychondritis* |

*Can commonly involve both veins and arteries.

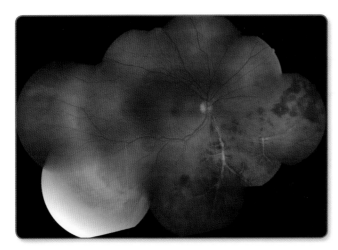

**Figure 52.1** Composite fundus photographs of the right eye. The optic nerve is hyperemic. The inferior vasculature resembles a 'frosted branch,' with inflammatory sheathing of the venous system. Hemorrhage traces the vascular pattern. There are numerous white centered hemorrhages in the inferior and nasal periphery.

# Final diagnosis: Behçet's disease

## Epidemiology/etiology

Behçet's disease is particularly common in people of Japanese, Southeast Asian, Middle Eastern, or Mediterranean descent. Men are affected more often than women. The mean age at onset is during the third decade of life. The cause of Behçet's disease is unknown, though genetic, environmental, and infectious factors have all been implicated. Ocular involvement is associated with HLA-B51.

## Symptoms and clinical findings

Patients typically present with blurred vision, eye pain, redness, and light sensitivity. Clinical diagnosis can be made based on the classic triad of recurrent aphthous oral ulcers, genital ulcers, and intraocular inflammation.

The hallmark ophthalmic finding of acute iritis with sterile hypopyon is present in about a third of cases. A mild vitritis is also typically

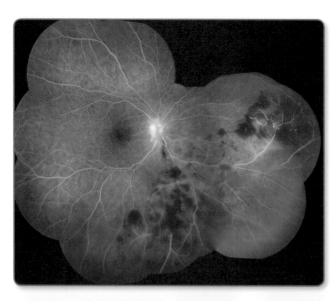

**Figure 52.2** Montage fluorescein angiogram of the right eye. The nerve leaks extensively. There is hypofluorescence due to blockage from retinal bleeding and due to ischemia from peripheral nonperfusion. Multiple retinal vessels leak dye, consistent with a vasculitic process.

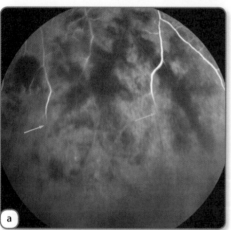

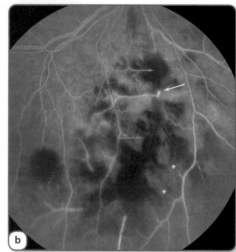

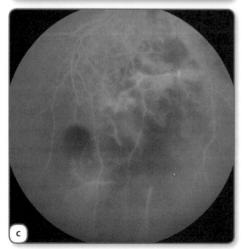

**Figure 52.3** Early (a) angiographic image reveals a 'leading edge' of dye (blue arrows) and distal nonperfusion. Mid-phase image demonstrates small vessel leakage (b). A ghost vessel can be seen (red arrows). Many of the vessels are pruned (asterisks). Early anastomoses can be seen (yellow arrow). (c) Late angiographic image reveals continued leakage from the smaller venules and persistent pruning and nonperfusion.

present. Retinal vasculitis, which may involve both arteries and veins, is the most common retinal manifestation. Unchecked, this can lead to retinal vascular occlusion, cystoid macular edema, ischemic retinal changes, and peripheral neovascularization. Deep yellowish-white retinal infiltrates can also be detected in some patients. These lesions appear similar to those seen with cat scratch disease.

Systemic vasculitis occurs in 25% of patients and may lead to granulomatous endocarditis, myocarditis, coronary arteritis, gastrointestinal ulceration, pulmonary arteritis with aneurysmal dilatation, and central nervous system vasculitis, the last of which has a 10% mortality rate.

## Treatment/prognosis/follow-up

Treatment usually requires high-dose systemic corticosteroids along with topical and periocular steroids. Cytotoxic agents, colchicine, and steroid-sparing immunomodulatory therapies such as cyclosporine or infliximab are often started to reduce recurrence of the disease and minimize steroid-induced contributions to cataract formation and glaucoma. Prior episodes of retinal ischemia may lead to peripheral neovascularization, which should be treated with laser photocoagulation. Without prompt and aggressive systemic treatment, visual prognosis is guarded as repeat episodes of inflammation can lead to optic and chorioretinal atrophy, pigment migration and subretinal fibrosis, macular ischemia, and peripheral ischemia with subsequent neovascular glaucoma.

# Further reading

Bonfioli AA, Orefice F. Behçet's disease. Semin Ophthalmol 2005; 20:199–206.

# Section 8

# Hereditary retinal and choroidal dystrophies

## How to approach a patient with insidious visual loss and poor night vision

| Identify the primary pathologic clinical finding(s) | | |
|---|---|---|
| In both eyes, there are bone spicules scattered throughout the nasal periphery. There are also curvilinear areas of atrophy in the temporal macula of each eye. | | |
| **Formulate a differential diagnosis** | | |
| **Most likely** | **Less likely** | **Least likely** |
| • Retinitis pigmentosa | • Prior retinal detachment, cancer-associated retinopathy, thioridazine toxicity, cone–rod dystrophy | • Vitamin A deficiency, syphilis, remote retinal vascular occlusion, Eales' disease, DUSN, AZOOR, congenital TORCH infection |
| **Query patient history** | | |
| • Does the patient have poor night vision? Any difficulty seeing in the dark?<br>• Is the patient on any medications?<br>• Does the patient have abnormal color vision?<br>• Is there a family history of retinal problems?<br>• Any difficulty hearing? | | |
| **Decide on ancillary diagnostic imaging** | | |
| Fundus photography is useful for patient education. Color vision testing and automated visual field testing can also provide important information. Optical coherence tomography is the best noninvasive ancillary test to evaluate the structure of the photoreceptors and RPE. Fundus autofluorescence (FAF) can also illustrate the health of the RPE. Fluorescein angiography should be obtained if the history and clinical appearance are consistent with a remote retinal vascular occlusion or ongoing retinal vasculitis. Full-field and multifocal ERG testing may be ultimately required to establish the diagnosis and quantify the degree of diminished photoreceptor function. | | |

## Ancillary diagnostic imaging interpretation

### Color photography

The media is clear in both eyes. The optic nerves are slightly pallorous. The retinal arteries are narrowed. Temporal to each fovea, there are large comma-shaped arcs of retina and RPE atrophy. The montage photos reveal bony spicules in the nasal periphery of each eye (**Figure 53.1**).

### Optical coherence tomography

The color maps reveal retinal thinning in a bull's-eye type pattern. The foveas are thinned with mild abnormality of the subfoveal IS/OS ellipsoid band. The immediate paracentral IS/OS ellipsoid bands are intact, but more peripherally there is complete loss of all outer retinal layers. The outer nuclear layer also attenuates outside fovea (**Figure 53.2**).

### Fundus autofluorescence

FAF clearly demonstrates a curvilinear area of RPE atrophy temporal to each fovea (**Figure 53.3**).

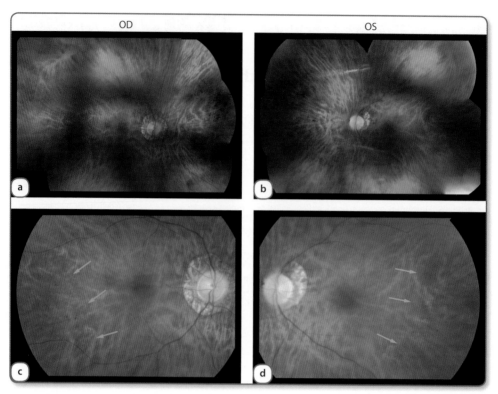

**Figure 53.1** Montage and posterior pole photographs of the right and left eyes. The arteries are narrowed and the discs are pallorous. There are areas of atrophy (blue arrows) in the temporal maculas. Bony spicules are noted in the periphery.

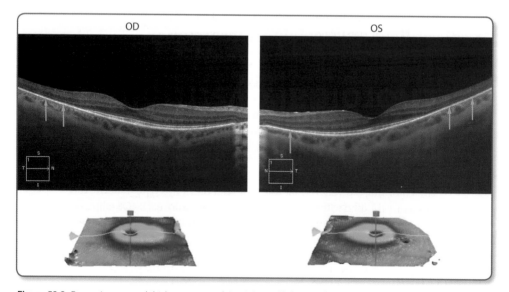

**Figure 53.2** B-scan images and thickness maps of the right and left eyes. There is mild foveal atrophy OU with abnormalities of the ellipsoid band. The outer nuclear layers taper and atrophy away from the fovea. There is loss of all outer retinal bands temporally in both eyes (blue arrows) and nasally OS. The thickness maps demonstrate a bull's-eye configuration.

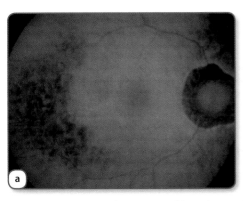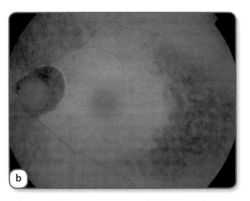

**Figure 53.3** Fundus autofluorescence of the right (a) and left (b) eyes demonstrates temporal and peripapillary hypoautofluorescence.

# Final diagnosis: retinitis pigmentosa, late onset

## Epidemiology/etiology

Retinitis pigmentosa is the name given to a series of retinal dystrophies that affect the photoreceptors and RPE. Half of the cases are sporadic, while the rest are passed in autosomal recessive (20%), autosomal dominant (20%), and X-linked (10%) fashion. Individuals with X-linked inheritance tend to present early, whereas those with autosomal dominant become symptomatic at an older age.

Multiple different mutations have been found to produce the retinitis pigmentosa (RP) phenotype (genetic heterogeneity). On the other hand, patients with similar mutations may demonstrate large variations in disease burden (pleiotropy). Regardless of the mutation involved, the final common process in patients with RP is apoptosis and death of the rod photoreceptors. Cone and RPE cells are frequently affected as well.

RP may be isolated to the eye or be part of a systemic process. Hearing loss is the most common association (Usher's syndrome).

RP is relatively common with a prevalence of 1/4000 worldwide. It typically affects teenagers and young adults in their second and third decades of life, but it also can be seen in very young patients and those in their 50s and 60s.

## Symptoms and clinical findings

Patients typically present with a slow onset of visual difficulties, which can include continuous photopsias, poor night vision, and difficulty driving, especially at dusk or in the fog and rain. Going from a light to dark room like in a movie theatre is especially problematic. In some cases, patients are unaware of any disability until formal testing is performed at a school or driving test examination. Younger children should have a formal hearing evaluation, given the association with Usher's syndrome. As the disease progresses, peripheral vision loss becomes symptomatic.

Slit lamp examination may reveal posterior subcapsular cataracts and mild anterior vitreous cells. The optic nerves often appear atrophic and pallorous. The retinal arteries are typically attenuated. Early on in the disease, the macula may appear normal. As time progresses, a bull's-eye type atrophic maculopathy may develop. Midperipheral RPE atrophy is also commonly noted. The classic finding is the appearance of pigmented bone spicules in a perivascular distribution in the peripheral retina.

Other less commonly seen findings include epiretinal membrane, cystoid macular edema, macular hole, yellow deposits (retinitis punctate albescens), vasoproliferative tumor and a Coat's-like telangiectasis.

Both eyes are typically affected in a symmetric pattern which, in general, is more indicative of a dystrophic, systemic, or toxic etiology rather than an inflammatory, infectious, or vascular cause.

## Treatment/prognosis/follow-up

For most patients, the disease slowly progresses over decades. In general, the later the onset of symptoms the more favorable the prognosis.

No treatment has been prospectively shown to significantly delay progression of the disease. High-dose vitamin A may slow the disease process by about 2% per year. This modest benefit must be weighed against the potential systemic risk of long-term high doses of vitamin A. Diamox, topical carbonic anhydrase inhibitors, or periocular steroids can be used to treat cystoid macular edema, if present. Cataract surgery is advisable in patients with significant posterior subcapsular cataract. Patients should be counseled against smoking. A diet rich in fish and green leafy vegetables is advisable. Sun-protection should be worn in bright conditions. Perhaps the most helpful option for patients with symptomatic RP is an early referral to a low vision specialist.

The FDA has recently approved a retina implant, the Argus II Retinal Prosthesis System, for patients with advanced RP. This implant may improve the ability of patients to perform their normal activities of daily living.

# Further reading

Berson EL, Rosner B, Sandberg MA, et al. A randomized trial of vitamin A and vitamin E supplementation for retinitis pigmentosa. Arch Ophthalmol 1993; 111:761–72.

Chang S, Vaccarella L, Olatunji S, et al. Diagnostic challenges in retinitis pigmentosa: genotypic multiplicity and phenotypic variability. Curr Genomics 2011; 12:267–75.

Rizzo S, Belting C, Cinelli L, et al. The Argus II retinal prosthesis: twelve-month outcomes from a single-study center. Am J Ophthalmol 2014;157:1282-90.

# 54

# Cone and cone–rod dystrophy

## How to approach a patient with insidious visual loss, poor color vision, and a bull's-eye maculopathy

| Identify the primary pathologic clinical finding(s) | | |
|---|---|---|
| In both eyes, there is a symmetric oval-shaped area of atrophy in a bull's-eye configuration. | | |
| **Formulate a differential diagnosis** | | |
| **Most likely** | **Less likely** | **Least likely** |
| • Cone dystrophy, cone–rod dystrophy | • Hydroxychloroquine toxicity, Stargardt's disease | • Benign concentric annular macular dystrophy, central areolar pigment epithelial dystrophy, atrophic Best's disease, retinitis pigmentosa |
| **Query patient history** | | |
| • Is the patient taking chloroquine or hydroxychloroquine?<br>• Does the patient have poor color vision?<br>• Does the patient have poor night vision?<br>• Does anyone in the family have poor vision that cannot be corrected with glasses? | | |
| **Decide on ancillary diagnostic imaging** | | |
| Fundus photography is useful for patient education. Color vision testing and automated visual field testing can also provide important information. Optical coherence tomography is the best noninvasive ancillary test to evaluate the structure of the photoreceptors and RPE. Fundus autofluorescence (FAF) can also illustrate the health of the RPE. Fluorescein angiography may show a 'silent choroid' in patients with Stargardt's disease, a finding which helps differentiate it from other causes of bull's-eye maculopathy. Full-field and multifocal ERG testing may ultimately be required to establish the diagnosis and quantify the degree of diminished photoreceptor function. | | |

## Ancillary diagnostic imaging interpretation

### Color photography

The media is clear in both eyes. The optic nerves appear unaffected, and the vasculature appears to be of normal caliber. In both eyes, there are oval-shaped areas of retinal atrophy centered upon the fovea. No yellow pisciform lesions are noted (**Figure 54.1**).

## Optical coherence tomography

In both eyes, the paracentral outer retina is abnormal with loss of the photoreceptor bands. The outer nuclear layers are attenuated. There are areas of pigment migration. The RPE appears relatively intact and choroid uninvolved (**Figure 54.2**).

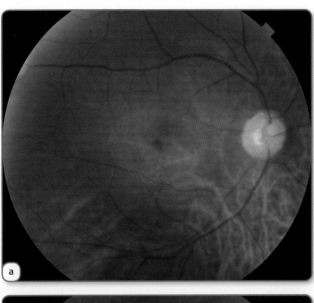

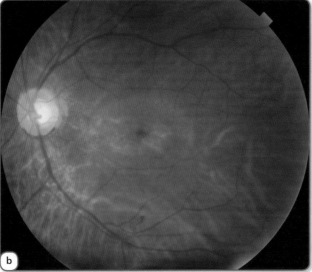

**Figure 54.1** Color photographs of the right (a) and left (b) eyes reveal a bull's-eye maculopathy OU.

## Fundus autofluorescence

FAF clearly demonstrates the donut-shaped area of atrophy. The rim of the lesion is hyperautofluorescent, while the central area is a mix of hyper- and hypoautofluorescence. The fovea appears relatively spared (**Figure 54.3**).

# Final diagnosis: cone dystrophy

## Epidemiology/etiology

The cone–rod dystrophies are a group of relatively rare disorders (1/40,000) that typically affect young adults in their first through third

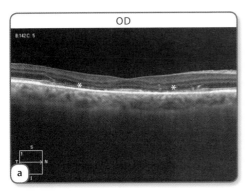
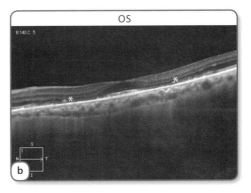

**Figure 54.2** Optical coherence tomographic images reveal blunted foveal contours in each eye. There is paracentral loss of the photoreceptor bands (asterisks) and attenuation of the outer nuclear layers. The left eye displays a 'flying saucer' sign that is also often seen in advanced hydroxychloroquine maculopathy. The RPE and choroid appear uninvolved.

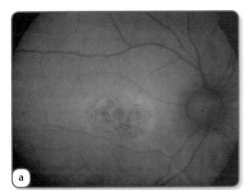
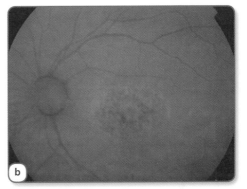

**Figure 54.3** Fundus autofluorescence highlights the area of atrophy in the right (a) and left (b) eyes. In each eye, there is a rim of hyperautofluorescence and mixed fluorescence within the lesion.

decades of life. They are characterized by a greater loss of cone function relative to rods. The etiology is unknown, though over 10 causative genetic mutations have been identified. Cone dystrophy may also arise as part of a syndrome such as Bardet-Biedl and spinocerebellar ataxia type 7.

## Symptoms and clinical findings

Patients typically present with a slow onset of visual difficulties, which can include photophobia, blurred vision, difficulty reading, and poor color discrimination. A central scotoma or area of distortion may be reported and patients may need to eccentrically fixate to view the smaller lines on the eye chart. In some cases, patients are unaware of any disability until formal testing is performed at a school or driving examination. As the disease progresses, rod function may also diminish, possibly to the point of symptomatic nyctalopia.

Slit lamp examination is unremarkable aside from rare anterior vitreous cells. The optic nerves may appear pale, especially on the temporal side, and the retinal vessels can be attenuated. Depending on the severity of disease, fundus examination can range from normal to a bull's-eye pattern of atrophy to widespread chorioretinal atrophy. ERG testing may demonstrate decreased bright flash amplitudes and diminished and slow flicker responses, indicative of cone dysfunction.

Hydroxychloroquine toxicity must be ruled out before considering other potential possibilities.

## Treatment/prognosis/follow-up

No treatment has been shown to slow progression of the disease. Patients should be counseled against smoking. A diet rich in fish and green leafy vegetables is advisable. Sun-protection should be worn in bright conditions. A referral to a low vision specialist is prudent.

# Further reading

Hamel CP. Cone rod dystrophies. Orphanet J Rare Dis 2007; 2:7.

Lima LH, Sallum JM, Spaide RF. Outer retina analysis by optical coherence tomography in cone-rod dystrophy patients. Retina 2013; 33:1877–80.

# 55

# Stargardt's disease

## How to approach a patient with insidious visual loss, a bull's-eye maculopathy, and yellow flecks in the retina

| Identify the primary pathologic clinical finding(s) | | |
|---|---|---|
| In both eyes, there are symmetric oval-shaped areas of atrophy centered upon the fovea. Yellow flecks are scattered around macula. | | |
| **Formulate a differential diagnosis** | | |
| Most likely | Less likely | Least likely |
| • Stargardt's disease | • Plaquenil toxicity, cone–rod dystrophy | • Benign concentric annular macular dystrophy, central areolar pigment epithelial dystrophy, atrophic Best's disease, retinitis punctata albescens, fundus albipunctatus |
| **Query patient history** | | |
| • Does the patient have any problems with color vision?<br>• Does the patient take any medications?<br>• Have they ever taken chloroquine or hydroxychloroquine?<br>• Does the patient have poor night vision?<br>• Is there a family history of poor vision that can't be corrected with glasses? | | |
| **Decide on ancillary diagnostic imaging** | | |
| Fundus photography is useful for patient education. Color vision testing and automated visual field testing can also provide important information. Optical coherence tomography is the best noninvasive ancillary test to evaluate the structure of the photoreceptors and RPE. Fundus autofluorescence (FAF) can assess the degree of RPE deterioration. It can also demonstrate peripapillary sparing which is a helpful diagnostic finding. Fluorescein angiography is essentially diagnostic if it reveals a 'silent' or 'dark' choroid. Full-field and multifocal ERG testing may be required if the diagnosis remains elusive after less invasive multimodality testing. | | |

## Ancillary diagnostic imaging interpretation

### Color photography

The media is clear in both eyes. The optic nerves appear unaffected, and the vasculature appears to be of normal caliber. In both eyes, there are symmetric oval-shaped areas of retina and RPE atrophy centered upon the fovea. These central areas have a metallic, polychromatic sheen. Yellow pisciform lesions are present (**Figure 55.1**).

### Optical coherence tomography

In both eyes, the retina is atrophic and extremely thinned at the fovea. The outer retina is abnormal with loss of the outer nuclear layer and all photoreceptor bands. The RPE line is also attenuated and in some areas only Bruch's membrane remains. There is increased light penetration into the choroid (**Figure 55.2**).

### Fundus autofluorescence

FAF clearly demonstrates the central area of retinal atrophy. The pisciform lesions are mostly hyperautofluorescent (**Figure 55.3**). The peripapillary areas appear uninvolved.

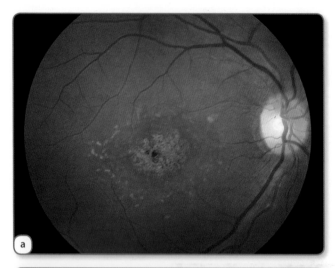

**Figure 55.1** Color photographs of the right (a) and left (b) eyes reveal numerous yellow flecks surrounding a central area of retina and RPE atrophy. There is a metallic sheen to the atrophy, quite prominent in the more affected left eye.

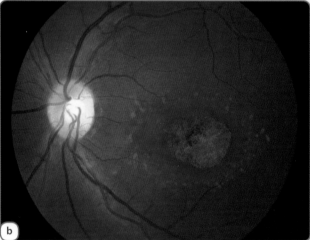

## Fluorescein angiography

The choroid is hypofluorescent (i.e. dark or silent). There is early central hyperfluorescence, consistent with a window defect (**Figure 55.4**).

## Final diagnosis: Stargardt's disease

### Epidemiology/etiology

Stargardt's disease typically affects school-aged children, teenagers, and young adults. There is no race or sex predilection. It is an autosomal recessive disorder caused by mutations in the *ABC4* gene. This gene encodes for proteins responsible for the active transport of various substrates between the RPE and outer retina. Within the Stargardt's spectrum, there is a significant variation in disease burden, related to mutation type and degree of residual *ABC4* activity.

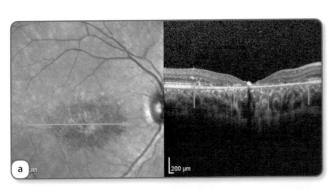

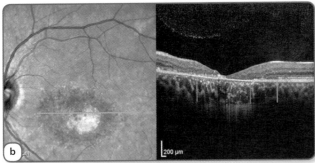

**Figure 55.2** Optical coherence tomographic images of the right (a) and left (b) eyes. The infrared photographs demonstrate a bull's-eye maculopathy. There is severe foveal thinning with near complete loss of all retinal layers. Outside the fovea, there is loss of the outer nuclear and photoreceptor layers (blue arrows). The RPE is also attenuated and Bruch's membrane is revealed in some areas (red arrows). The blue arrows point to a transition point between relatively normal photoreceptors and outer retinal atrophy. There is increased light penetration into the choroid. There is a hyper-reflective lesion in the fovea of the right eye of uncertain significance.

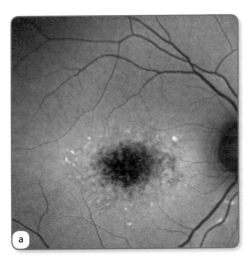

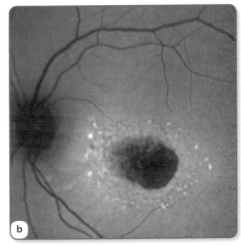

**Figure 55.3** Fundus autofluorescence images demonstrate central hypofluorescence that corresponds to the areas of retina and RPE atrophy seen clinically and tomographically. Many of the flecks are hyperautofluorescent, reflective of lipofuscin accumulation.

## Symptoms and clinical findings

Patients typically present with a slow onset of visual difficulties, which can include blurred vision, difficulty reading, central scotomas, and poor color discrimination. In some cases, patients are unaware of any disability until formal testing is performed at a school or driving examination.

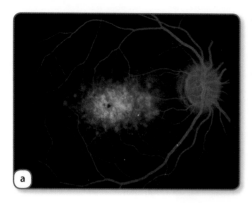
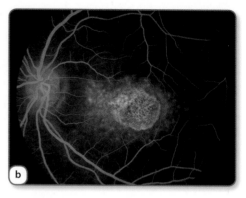

**Figure 55.4** Fluorescein angiographic images of the right (a) and left (b) eyes demonstrate a 'silent' or 'dark' choroid due to blocking of normal choroidal fluorescence by lipofuscin-filled RPE cells. The central macula is hyperfluorescent, a window defect from retina and RPE atrophy. In the left eye, a few larger choroidal vessels can be appreciated within the bed of atrophy, suggestive of RPE and choriocapillaris atrophy.

Visual acuity at presentation can range from 20/20 to levels consistent with legal blindness. These patients do not typically report nyctalopia.

Slit lamp examination is unremarkable. Depending on the severity of disease, fundus examination can range from normal to mild pigment epithelial change to a bull's-eye maculopathy. The disease can spread in a centrifugal fashion and result in widespread chorioretinal atrophy. The classic findings consist of yellow pisciform lesions scattered throughout the macula and periphery. These flecks represent lipofuscin accumulation within the RPE. The flecks are typically hyperautofluorescent. Another common feature in Stargardt's disease is relative sparing of the peripapillary retina. Dark choroid is also seen in a majority of patients, and is the result of blockage of choroidal fluorescence by lipofuscin-rich RPE cells.

## Treatment/prognosis/follow-up

The prognosis for these patients is typically poor. In general, younger age and worse vision at presentation are correlated with poorer outcomes. Late-onset Stargardt's disease has also been described. These patients have better visual acuity, higher likelihood of foveal sparing, and slower rates of progression.

No treatment has been shown to slow progression of the disease. Patients should be counseled against smoking. A diet rich in fish and green leafy vegetables is advisable, and sun-protection is prudent. There is no role for high-dose vitamin intake. Gene therapy may eventually play a role in the management of patients with more severe disease burden.

## Further reading

Rotenstreich Y, Fishman GA, Anderson RJ. Visual acuity loss and clinical observations in a large series of patients with Stargardt disease. Ophthalmology 2003; 110:1151–8.

Westeneng-van Haaften SC, Boon CJ, Cremers FP, et al. Clinical and genetic characteristics of late-onset Stargardt's disease. Ophthalmology 2012; 119:1199–210.

## How to approach a young patient with insidious visual loss and yellow-orange macular lesions

| Identify the primary pathologic clinical finding(s) | | |
|---|---|---|
| In the right eye, there is an irregular area of pigment change that is rimmed by orange-appearing dots. The left eye has a similar appearing oval-shaped area of RPE change with an orange outline. | | |
| **Formulate a differential diagnosis** | | |
| **Most likely** | **Less likely** | **Least likely** |
| • Autosomal recessive bestrophinopathy (ARB) | • Chronic central serous retinopathy, Stargardt's disease, 'scrambled' or atrophic Best's disease | • Macular dystrophy associated with maternally inherited diabetes and deafness, multifocal pattern dystrophy, cone–rod dystrophy, persistent placoid maculopathy, syphilitic chorioretinitis |
| **Query patient history** | | |
| • Is there a family history of vision not correctable with glasses?<br>• Can the patient see in the dark?<br>• Does the patient have normal color vision?<br>• Any family history of hearing loss? | | |
| **Decide on ancillary diagnostic imaging** | | |
| Fundus photography is useful for patient education. Optical coherence tomography is the best noninvasive ancillary test to evaluate the structure of the photoreceptors and RPE. Fundus autofluorescence can also illustrate the health of the RPE and may be diagnostic in patients with typical Best's or ARB. Fluorescein angiography may reveal smokestack leaks or an expanding dot of leakage, which can be suggestive of central serous retinopathy. Electrophysiologic testing consisting of full-field ERG, multifocal ERG, and EOG may ultimately be required to establish the diagnosis and quantify the extent of diminished photoreceptor and RPE function. | | |

## Ancillary diagnostic imaging interpretation

### Color photography

The media is clear in both eyes. The optic nerves and retinal vasculature appear normal.

In the right eye, the fovea appears atrophic and yellow lutein pigment is visible. There is a V-shaped area of retinal and RPE change. There is an orangish outline surrounding this abnormal area. Multiple orange dots or flecks reside in this border. There is a suggestion of a 'gutter' due to past dependent subretinal fluid (**Figure 56.1**).

The left eye also has an atrophic appearing fovea. There is a horizontal oval-shaped area of RPE and retinal atrophy temporal to the fovea that again has an orange outline.

### Optical coherence tomography

A horizontal B scan through the fovea of the right eye reveals a low-lying and diffuse enlargement of the space between the RPE and outer

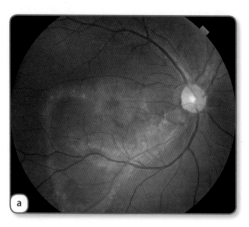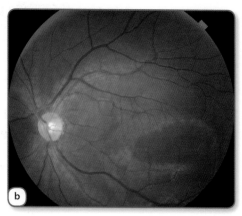

**Figure 56.1** Color photographs of the right (a) and left (b) eyes demonstrate irregular-shaped areas of retina and RPE change. A rim of orange surrounds the disturbed areas.

retina (vitelliform space). There is hyper-reflective material within the fluid filled space, best seen nasal to the fovea (**Figure 56.2a**).

Optical coherence tomography of the left eye also demonstrates subretinal fluid with an irregular enlargement of the vitelliform space. The photoreceptor outer segments have been disrupted (**Figure 56.2b**).

## Fundus autofluorescence

The outlines defining the irregular areas of atrophy are clearly hyperautofluorescent. The areas of atrophy are mildly hypoautofluorescent. There is mixed autofluorescence in the foveal regions (**Figure 56.3**).

## Fluorescein angiography

An early angiographic image of the left eye demonstrates a hyperfluorescent border (window defect). The nasal edge of the lesion stains with fluorescence as the study progresses. No definite leak is noted in either eye (**Figure 56.4**).

## Final diagnosis: ARB

### Epidemiology/etiology

Mutations in the *BEST1* gene lead to a group of rare, hereditary retinal pigment epithelial dystrophies. This gene encodes for a transmembrane protein important in maintaining fluid and ion transport between the RPE and outer retina. Dysfunction of this protein leads to the accumulation of lipofuscin in the RPE and in the potential space between the RPE and retina.

Best vitelliform macular dystrophy is the most common *BEST1*-related retinal dystrophy. These patients develop classic 'egg yolk' or vitelliform lesions that evolve in appearance over time. Typical Best's disease is passed in an autosomal dominant fashion. It can be

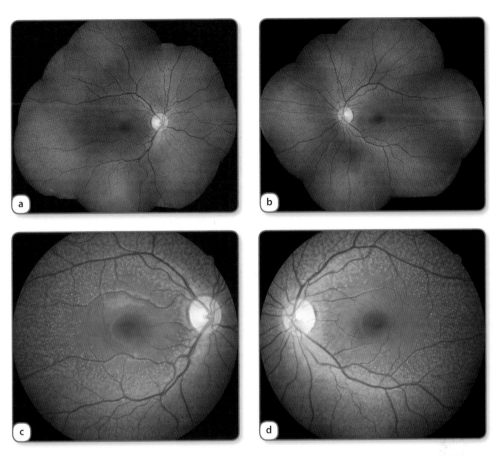

**Figure 57.2** Color montage photos and posterior pole images of the right and left eyes of the older sister (aged 13 years). The flecks are lesser in number and are noted just inside of the vascular arcades. Outside the macula, a diffuse epithelialopathy is again seen. By courtesy of Dr Sam Yang, Walnut Creek, CA, USA.

Biomicroscopy reveals the presence of numerous yellow-white, polymorphous lesions throughout the posterior pole, midperiphery, and periphery; sparing of the fovea and papillomacular bundle is typical. Secondary RPE changes are usually absent.

On OCT, the flecks appear as hyper-reflective deposits located posterior to the IS/OS ellipsoid layer/outer photoreceptor tips. The external limiting membrane and RPE are not involved. FA may reveal irregular, diffuse hyperfluorescence that is suggestive of an underlying abnormality of the RPE. Hyperfluorescence on angiography does not seem to correspond to the location of the flecks. The flecks appear hyperautofluorescent, suggesting the presence of lipofuscin.

Electrophysiology studies should be performed in order to rule out other possible diagnoses. The photopic and scotopic ERG in benign familial flecked retina are typically normal, as are other tests such as the electro-oculogram and visual evoked potential.

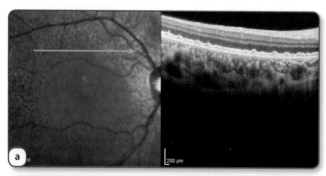

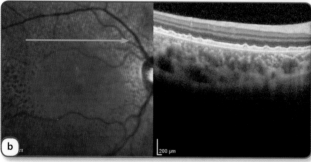

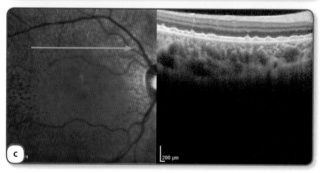

**Figure 57.3** Optical coherence tomography cross-sectional image through the superior macula of the older sister. The flecks reside in the deep retina and irregularly elevate the IS/OS ellipsoid band. By courtesy of Dr Sam Yang, Walnut Creek, CA, USA.

## Treatment/prognosis/follow-up

Over time, the flecks may become less discrete and more confluent. They do not typically cause secondary changes to the overlying retina.

The condition is considered to be benign, and no treatment in necessary.

## Further reading

Audo I, Tsang SH, Fu AD, et al. Autofluorescence imaging in a case of benign familial fleck retina. Arch Ophthalmol 2011; 125:714–15.

Isaacs TW, McAllister IL, Wade MS. Benign fleck retina. Br J Ophthalmol 1996; 80:267–9.

Sabel Aish SF, Dajani B. Benign familial fleck retina. Br J Ophthalmol 1980; 64:652–9.

Sergouniotis PI, Davidson AE, Mackay DS, et al. Biallelic mutations in PLA2G5, ncoding group V phospholipase A$_2$, cause benign fleck retina. Am J Hum Genet 2011; 89:782–91.

## How to approach a patient with a depigmented fundus

| Identify the primary pathologic clinical finding(s) | | |
|---|---|---|
| In both eyes, there is a lack of pigment in the retinal pigment epithelium and choroid. Choroidal detail is clearly seen. | | |
| **Formulate a differential diagnosis** | | |
| Most likely | Less likely | Least likely |
| • Oculocutaneous albinism | • X-linked ocular albinism, choroideremia, thioridazine toxicity | • Normal variant (blonde fundus), end-stage posterior uveitis, aniridia |
| **Query patient history** | | |
| • Is there a history of albinism?<br>• Does the patient dye their hair?<br>• Is there a history of unusual eye movements or of patching as a child?<br>• Any problems with bleeding or easy bruising?<br>• Any problems with recurrent infections? | | |
| **Decide on ancillary diagnostic imaging** | | |
| Fundus photography is useful for patient education. Optical coherence tomography (OCT) may demonstrate foveal hypoplasia or macular schisis. Fundus autofluorescein and fuorescein angiography are unlikely to be helpful. | | |

## Ancillary diagnostic imaging interpretation

### Color photography

The media is clear in both eyes. The optic nerves appear unaffected. There is a near-total absence of pigmentation in the fundus of both eyes, allowing clear visualization of choroidal detail (**Figure 58.1**).

### Optical coherence tomography

Right eye: The foveal depression is absent. The inner retinal layers (inner limiting membrane to the outer plexiform layers) do not taper toward the fovea as they normally do. The outer retina appears intact. The 'inverse umbo,' the increase in height of the IS/OS junction underneath the fovea, is missing (**Figure 58.2**).

Left eye: Again, the foveal depression is absent and the inner retina remains thickened over the anatomical fovea. There is a schisis-like change in the inner nuclear layer and a large cyst within the outer nuclear layer. Unlike the right eye, the left eye demonstrates outer retinal abnormalities as well. The outer nuclear layer attenuates and the photoreceptor bands are missing outside the fovea. The thickness map nicely illustrates the perifoveal thinning.

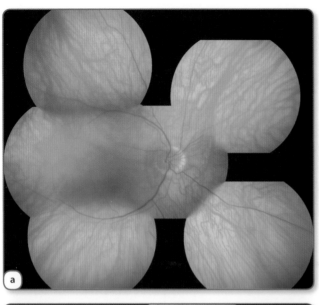

**Figure 58.1** Montage photographs of the right (a) and left (b) eyes reveal near complete depigmentation of the fundus. Choroidal detail is easily seen. By courtesy of Dr Nadia Waheed, MD, Boston, MA, USA.

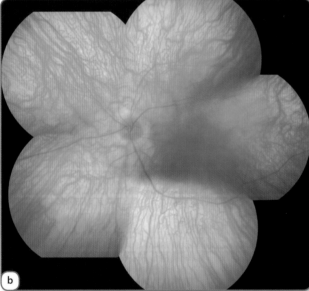

# Final diagnosis: oculocutaneous albinism

## Epidemiology/etiology

Albinism results from a disruption in melanin production or metabolism. It may be seen in all racial groups, though it is most common in African American populations.

Albinism can be divided into two categories: ocular and oculocutaneous. Ocular albinism is limited to the eye and may be transmitted in an X-linked or autosomal recessive fashion.

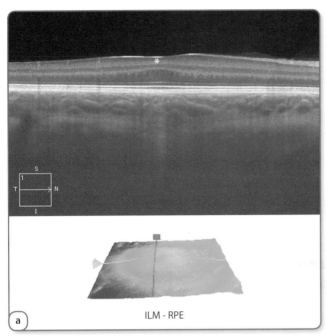

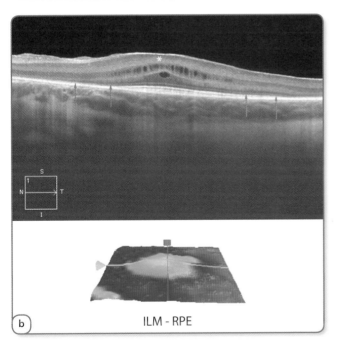

**Figure 58.2** Optical coherence tomographic images and thickness maps of the right and left eyes. In both eyes, the highly reflective internal limiting membrane (IML) crosses over the fovea. Inner retinal layers such as the ganglion cell, inner plexiform, and inner nuclear layer also endure across the fovea (asterisks). The 'inverse umbo' is absent OU. The retinal pigment epithelium (RPE) appears intact though there is greater visibility into the choroid and sclera, likely due to the lack of reflective pigment within the RPE and choroid. The left eye demonstrates a schisis-type change within the nuclear layers. The left also reveals severe loss of the photoreceptor bands outside the fovea (red arrows). By courtesy of Dr Nadia Waheed, MD, Boston, MA, USA.

Patients with oculocutaneous albinism have both eye and skin involvement. It is transmitted in an autosomal recessive fashion. There are numerous types of oculocutaneous albinism, the most well known are type I (tyrosinase negative) and type II (tyrosinase positive). Patients with type 1 albinism have a complete absence of skin and ocular pigmentation. There are two types of albinism that are linked with serious systemic abnormalities: Chediak–Higashi and Hermansky–Pudlak syndromes.

## Symptoms and clinical findings

Patients typically come to medical attention at a young age. They may present with poor vision or after failing a school eye examination. Furthermore, unstable or crossed eyes may be noted by the parents. Children may also complain of severe light sensitivity, requiring sunglasses even in low-light conditions.

Clinical findings may include poor stereopsis, a head tilt, pendular nystagmus, and strabismus. Visual acuity may range from normal to levels consistent with legal blindness. Slit lamp examination may reveal iris transillumination defects. Fundus examination is remarkable for loss of the foveal pit and retinal vessels that may course through the typically avascular foveal zone. The peripheral fundus is generally depigmented. Of note, female carriers may display variable peripheral retinal pigmentary disturbances, variants that have been referred to as 'mud-slung' or 'bear track' pigmentation.

OCT has become a crucial ancillary test in the evaluation of these patients, with findings that are consistent with macular hypoplasia and/or macular schisis.

Patients with Chediak–Higashi syndrome suffer from recurrent pyogenic infections, whereas those afflicted with Hermansky–Pudlak syndrome are prone to repeated bleeding episodes. Consultation with a hematologist/oncologist specialist is advisable.

## Treatment/prognosis/follow-up

Refractive errors, strabismus and amblyopia, and nystagmus should be managed by a skilled pediatric ophthalmologist. No specific medical therapy is available. A low-vision evaluation is recommended.

## Further reading

Chong GT, Farsiu S, Freedman SF, et al. Abnormal foveal morphology in ocular albinism imaged with spectral-domain optical coherence tomography. Arch Ophthalmol 2009; 127:37–44.

Costa DL, Huang SJ, Donsoff IM, Yannuzzi LA. X-linked ocular albinism: fundus of a heterozygous female. Retina 2003; 23:410–11.

## How to approach a patient with bilateral macular schisis

| Identify the primary pathologic clinical finding(s) | | |
| --- | --- | --- |
| There is a spoke-like cystic appearance to the fovea in both eyes. | | |
| **Formulate a differential diagnosis** | | |
| Most likely | Less likely | Least likely |
| • X-linked juvenile retinoschisis (XJR) | • Oculocutaneous albinism, X-linked albinism, niacin toxicity | • Autosomal recessive bestrophinopathy, optic pit maculopathy, chronic central serous retinopathy, retinitis pigmentosa |
| **Query patient history** | | |
| • Any family members with poor vision uncorrectable by glasses?<br>• Are affected family members all men?<br>• Is there difficulty in seeing in the dark?<br>• Is there a history of taking high dose vitamins? | | |
| **Decide on ancillary diagnostic imaging** | | |
| Fundus photography is useful for patient education. Optical coherence tomography may demonstrate macular schisis and be used to track the response to topical or oral medications. Despite the presence of numerous cystic cavities, fluorescein angiography may not demonstrate petaloid leakage (Box 59.1). If the diagnosis remains in doubt, negative-shaped ERG responses may help pinpoint the diagnosis. | | |

## Ancillary diagnostic imaging interpretation

### Color photography

The media is clear in both eyes. The optic nerves appear unaffected. There are radial-oriented retinal striae pointing at the fovea in both eyes. Stellate cystic cavities are seen bilaterally (**Figure 59.1**).

### Optical coherence tomography

The infrared photographs demonstrate a bull's-eye pattern with obvious cystic change. Horizontal cross sections reveal a severe schisis-type change. It appears to predominantly involve the inner nuclear layer. The outer retinal layers are compressed by the large cystic cavities (**Figure 59.2**).

## Final diagnosis: XJR

### Epidemiology/etiology

XJR is a rare genetic disorder affecting 1/5000 to 1/25,000 children. It is due to a mutation in the *XLRS1* gene, located on the X-chromosome. It encodes for the protein retinoschisin that is crucial in maintaining cellular adhesion within the inner nuclear layer, as well as synaptic connections between the bipolar cells and the photoreceptors. Due to X-linked inheritance, men are primarily affected.

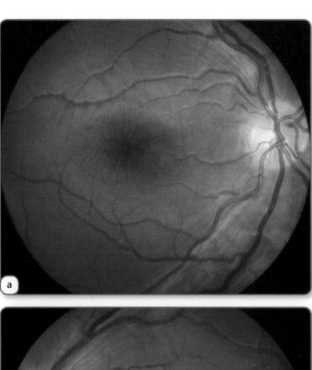

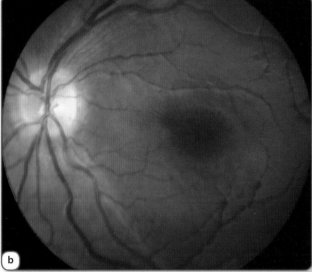

**Figure 59.1** Color photographs of the (a) right and (b) left eyes demonstrate bilateral macular cystoid cavities.

## Symptoms and clinical findings

Patients typically present at a young age. They complain of difficulty reading, blurred distance vision, or are referred after failing a school eye examination. Visual acuity at presentation can range from normal to levels consistent with legal blindness. These patients are frequently found to be hyperopic. Strabismus and nystagmus are not uncommon.

Stellate cystic foveal changes are noted in 100% of patients with typical sex-linked retinoschisis. Peripheral retinoschisis is found in half of these patients and vitreous veils and inner layer holes are often

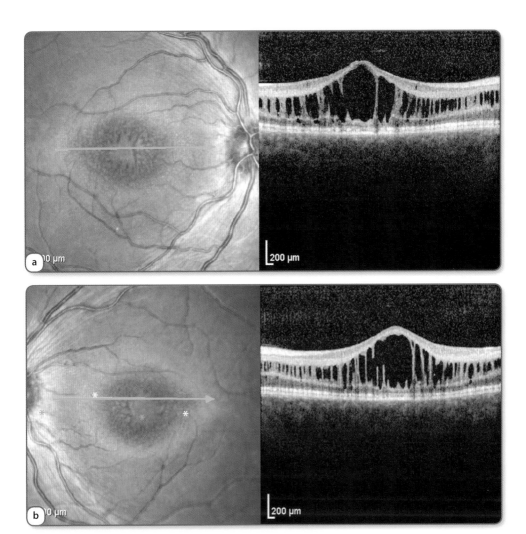

**Figure 59.2** Optical coherence tomographic images of the (a) right and (b) left macula. Infrared photos demonstrate a bull's eye type maculopathy. Cystic cavities are clearly highlighted. Horizontal B scans reveal large schisis-type cystoid macular edema. The cystic structures appear to be compressing the ganglion cell layers anteriorly and the outer plexiform and nuclear layers posteriorly. It is difficult to judge the status of the photoreceptor bands as thin strands of bridging retinal tissue (probable stretched Muller cells) cast a narrow shadow posteriorly.

present. Vessels that transverse the schisis cavities can tear, leading to vitreous hemorrhage. In fact, the most common etiology of vitreous hemorrhage in young boys is XJR.

## Treatment/prognosis/follow-up

Topical and oral carbonic anhydrase inhibitors may be used to decrease the size of macular schisis cavities, though the chronic use of these medicines has not been shown to alter the ultimate course of the disease. Surgery is advisable in patients who develop rhegmatogenous or tractional retinal detachment. Chronic vitreous hemorrhage may also necessitate vitrectomy. Prophylactic scatter laser has not shown to be beneficial in preventing retinal detachment or vitreous hemorrhage. Low vision referral should be made early in the disease course.

---

### Conditions associated with nonleaking cystoid macular edema

- Niacin toxicity
- Taxane-based chemotherapy toxicity
- X-linked juvenile retinoschisis
- Goldmann-Favre and other forms of retinitis pigmentosa
- Epiretinal membrane/vitreomacular traction syndrome

---

## Further reading

Salvatore S, Fishman GA, Genead MA. Treatment of cystic macular lesions in hereditary retinal dystrophies. Surv Ophthalmol 2013; 58:560–84.

# Section 9

# Neoplasms

# How to approach a patient with minimally elevated or flat pigmented choroidal lesion

| Identify the primary pathologic clinical finding(s) | | |
|---|---|---|
| There is a flat appearing, pigmented, choroidal lesion often with feathered edges located anywhere within the fundus (Figure 60.1). | | |
| **Formulate a differential diagnosis** | | |
| Most likely | Less likely | Least likely |
| • Choroidal nevus, choroidal freckle | • Choroidal melanoma, choroidal hemangioma, congenital hyperplasia of the retinal pigment epithelium | • Choroidal metastasis, choroidal hemorrhage, subretinal hemorrhage |
| **Query patient history** | | |
| • Is there any effect on vision?<br>• Has this lesion ever been noted during prior examinations?<br>• Is there any history of systemic malignancy? Family history of cancer?<br>• Has there been any recent ocular surgery or trauma? | | |
| **Decide on ancillary diagnostic imaging** | | |
| Fundus photography, fluorescein angiography, B-scan ultrasonography, fundus autofluorescence, and optical coherence tomography can all be useful to clarify the diagnoses being considered. | | |

# Ancillary diagnostic imaging interpretation

## Color photography

Fundus photography is helpful to document the appearance of the lesion so that future changes can be more easily detected in comparison to clinical examination and fundus drawings alone (**Figure 60.1**). This imaging modality is particularly sensitive to lesion growth in basal dimensions. Three illustrative examples show the varied clinical appearance to this condition.

## Optical coherence tomography

Optical coherence tomography (OCT), particularly with enhanced depth imaging modalities, can be useful to image the surface of these lesions to detect any associated subclinical features such as subretinal fluid, photoreceptor loss, and RPE irregularities. OCT is also helpful to demonstrate the presence or absence of any shallow elevation associated with the lesion and to measure lesion dimensions, particularly in smaller lesions where the sensitivity of traditional ultrasound is poor (**Figure 60.2**).

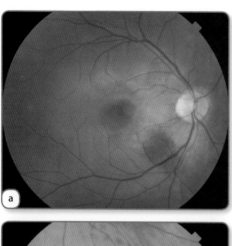

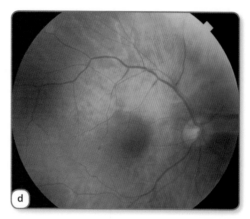

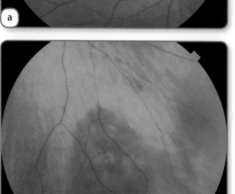

**Figure 60.1** Fundus photographs of choroidal nevi. Three examples of choroidal nevi are shown (a–c), each with a slightly different appearance but all are darkly pigmented, small, well circumscribed with feathered edges, and with no or minimal elevation. There is a typical choroidal nevus located in the inferonasal macula (a), one located in the fovea (b), and one located in the midperiphery with overlying drusen (c).

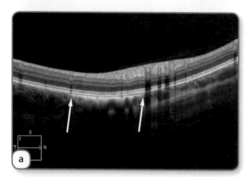

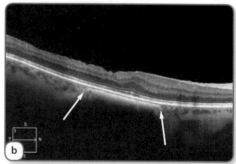

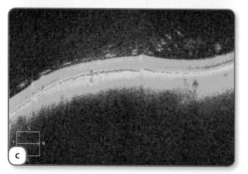

**Figure 60.2** Optical coherence tomography of choroidal nevi (corresponding to Figure 60.1a–c). Optical coherence tomography (OCT) shows hyper-reflectivity at the level of the superficial choroid in flat nevi, which obscures the surrounding choroidal vasculature (a, b, between arrows). OCT is also able to confirm slight elevation in a nevus that was thought to be minimally elevated clinically (c).

## Fluorescein angiography

Fluorescein angiography may be useful to evaluate for an internal vascular circulation, which would not be expected in a choroidal nevus. It also can detect associated choroidal neovascularization. Complete blockage of fluorescence suggests a hemorrhage (**Figure 60.3**).

## Fundus autofluorescence

Fundus autofluorescence shows a pattern of hypoautofluorescence in the location of a pigmented lesion such as a choroidal nevus. The presence of overlying drusen may elicit mild hyperfluorescence while the presence of overlying lipofuscin typically elicits bright hyperfluorescence (**Figure 60.4**).

## B-scan ultrasound

Ultrasound is particularly useful to measure and detect changes in choroidal lesion height (**Figure 60.5**).

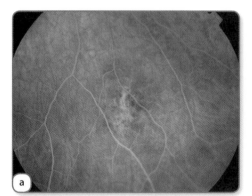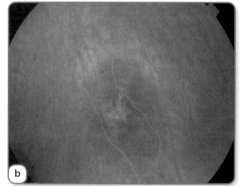

**Figure 60.3** Fluorescein angiography of a choroidal nevus (corresponding to Figures 60.1c and 60.2c). Early (a) and late (b) frames show generalized hypofluorescence in the region of the nevus (better visualized in b) along with early overlying hyperfluorescence corresponding to drusen.

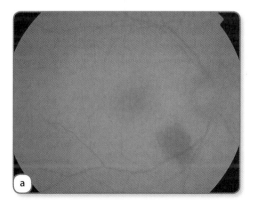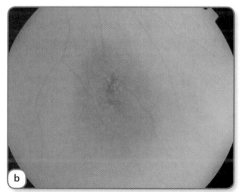

**Figure 60.4** Fundus autofluorescence of choroidal nevi (corresponding to Figure 60.1a and c). (a) There is hypoautofluorescence in the area of the choroidal nevi. Overlying drusen (b) exhibit mild hyperautofluorescence.

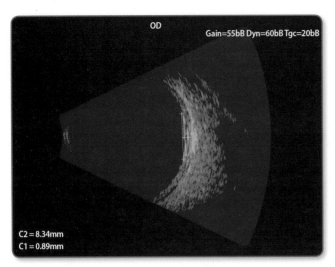

**Figure 60.5** B-scan ultrasound of choroidal nevi (corresponding to Figure 60.1c). Ultrasound demonstrates the ability to precisely measure basal diameter (8.34 mm) and height (0.89 mm) in a minimally elevated choroidal nevus

# Final diagnosis: choroidal nevus

## Epidemiology/etiology

Choroidal nevi are a common clinical finding, technically a benign melanocytic tumor, usually detected as an incidental finding in individuals during routine ophthalmic examination. Their prevalence is about 6.5% in Caucasian individuals (Sumich), and less prevalent in darkly pigmented individuals. The natural history of these lesions is of relative stability but minimal or slow growth in benign lesions is possible. There is a rare risk of malignant transformation into malignant melanoma of approximately 1 in 8845 (Singh), which underscores the importance of routine surveillance.

## Symptoms and clinical findings

Most patients with choroidal nevi are asymptomatic although vision can rarely be affected either as decreased central acuity or an isolated visual field defect. In general, nevi are flat, darkly pigmented, relatively well circumscribed, and isolated, although multiple nevi can be present. They are typically small in size (<10 mm across), flat or minimally elevated (<2 mm), and located toward the posterior fundus. Associated clinical features include surface drusen, RPE hyperplasia, or other irregularities and rarely subretinal fluid or choroidal neovascularization.

## Treatment/prognosis/follow-up

Clearly benign nevi should be monitored annually, although if being diagnosed for the first time, shorter follow-up intervals initially are prudent. If there is a question as to the benign nature of a suspected choroidal nevus (See Box below), diagnostic testing should be

---

## Clinical features favoring benign nature of a melanocytic choroidal lesion

Height <2.0 mm
Lack of lipofuscin
Presence of drusen
Lack of growth
Smaller overall dimensions
Lack of overlying subretinal fluid
Lack of symptoms
Not close to optic nerve

---

performed to document the current appearance and evaluate for features more typical of malignant lesions such as choroidal melanoma. Close follow-up, typically at an interval of 2–3 months is indicated in suspicious lesions to detect any lesion changes. In rare cases where there is secondary subretinal fluid or choroidal neovascularization associated with a choroidal nevus, treatment may be indicated, which can include focal laser or anti-VEGF therapy.

## Further reading

Singh AD, Kalyani P, Topham A. Estimating the risk of malignant transformation of a choroidal nevus. Ophthalmology 2005; 112:1784–9.
Sumich P, Mitchell P, Wang JJ. Choroidal nevi in a white population: the Blue Mountains Eye Study. Arch Ophthalmol 1998; 116:645–50.

# Choroidal melanoma

## How to approach a patient with an elevated, pigmented subretinal lesion

| Identify the primary pathologic clinical finding(s) | | |
|---|---|---|
| There is a large, darkly pigmented mass lesion located underneath the retina associated with orange pigment and a surrounding serous retinal detachment (**Figure 61.1a**). | | |
| **Formulate a differential diagnosis** | | |
| **Most likely** | **Less likely** | **Least likely** |
| • Choroidal melanoma, choroidal nevus | • Melanocytoma, choroidal hemangioma, choroidal metastasis, choroidal or retinal pigment epithelium (RPE) hemorrhage, retinal detachment, peripheral exudative hemorrhagic chorioretinopathy | • Subretinal hemorrhage, combined hamartoma, retinal macroaneurysm, posterior scleritis |
| **Query patient history** | | |
| • Does the patient have any history of systemic malignancy? Is there a family history of cancer?<br>• Is there any associated visual defect?<br>• If the lesion has been noted previously, has it changed in size or appearance since the initial evaluation?<br>• Are there any other associated symptoms such as eye pain? | | |
| **Decide on ancillary diagnostic imaging** | | |
| Clinical examination is the key to making the correct diagnosis, but ancillary diagnostic testing is also essential. A- and B-scan ultrasounds are important to measure the lesion height and to detect characteristic acoustic patterns. Ultrasound may also detect associated subclinical subretinal fluid. Fluorescein angiography (FA) is used to identify characteristic angiographic leakage patterns. Depending on the location of the lesion, optical coherence tomography (OCT) can be more sensitive than B-scan ultrasound to detect cystoid macular edema or subretinal fluid in the macula. | | |

## Ancillary diagnostic imaging interpretation

### Optical coherence tomography

OCT is very sensitive to detect even small amounts of subretinal fluid that may extend into the macula due to an associated serous retinal detachment in the presence of a choroidal melanoma (**Figure 61.2**). Associated CME may also be present. OCT can also be used to scan areas overlying the lesion to detect cystoid macular edema (CME) and/ or subretinal fluid.

### Fluorescein angiography

FA may display various characteristic features in choroidal melanoma including a secondary or intrinsic circulation of the tumor, extensive hyperfluorescence of the tumor itself, and numerous pinpoint areas of leakage (**Figure 61.3**).

### Indocyanine green angiography

Indocyanine green angiography can be very useful to evaluate for choroidal hemangioma, if that is being considered in the differential diagnosis.

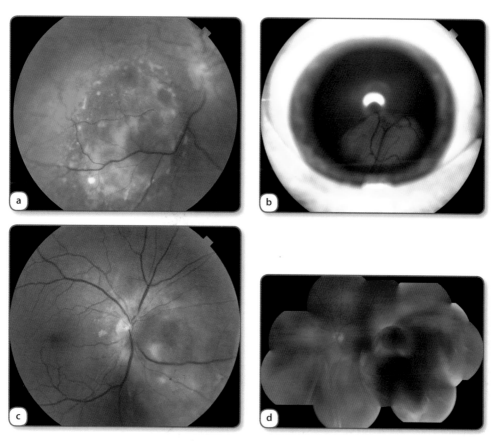

**Figure 61.1** Color photographs illustrating the variable appearance of choroidal melanomas (a–d). (a) A choroidal melanoma in the macula with overlying lipofuscin and shallow surrounding serous retinal detachment. (b) A large, anterior, amelanotic choroidal melanoma visible from an external view of the eye. (c) A peripapillary choroidal melanoma. (d) A very large, darkly pigmented choroidal melanoma located in the inferotemporal periphery associated with a large overlying serous retinal detachment (most prominent inferonasal).

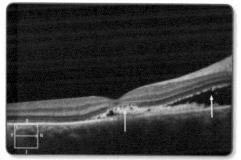

**Figure 61.2** Optical coherence tomography of associated subretinal fluid with choroidal melanoma (corresponding to Figure 61.1d). Subretinal fluid extending into the macula (white arrow) is present along with hyper-reflective deposits underneath the fovea (yellow arrow).

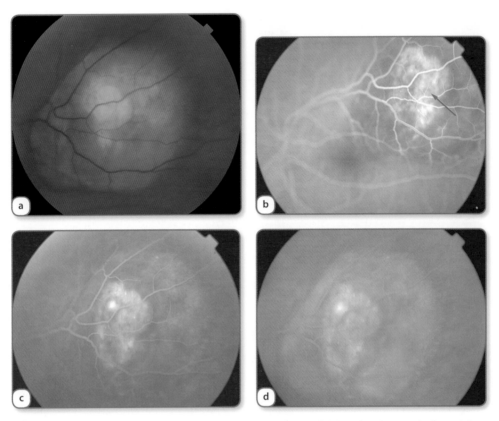

**Figure 61.3** Fluorescein angiographic features of choroidal melanoma (a–d). (a) Fundus photograph of a partially amelanotic choroidal melanoma. (b) Early phase fluorescein angiogram demonstrates generalized blockage from the lesion and an internal circulation located centrally (red arrow). Mid (c) and late (d) recirculation phase angiograms demonstrate decreasing hyperfluorescence of the internal circulation, increasing hyperfluorescence along the remaining portion of the tumor, and numerous pinpoint areas of hyperfluorescence, particularly on the right-most edge of the tumor.

## Fundus autofluorescence

The presence of lipofuscin overlying a suspected choroidal melanoma can be confirmed by its prominent hyperautoflourescence (**Figure 61.4**).

## Color photography

Serial color photographs are extremely useful to document any changes in tumor appearance or basal dimensions over time, which may help to confirm the diagnosis of choroidal melanoma compared to other similar lesions that would not be expected to grow.

## A- and B-scan ultrasonongraphy

Ultrasound is the most useful ancillary diagnostic test in the evaluation of a choroidal tumor. Characteristic features in choroidal melanoma include low-to-medium internal reflectivity, a silent internal acoustic zone within the tumor, and loss of the choroid in the region of the tumor (**Figure 61.5**).

# Final diagnosis: choroidal melanoma

## Epidemiology/etiology

Choroidal melanoma is the most common primary intraocular malignant tumor with an incidence of approximately five to six occurrences per 1 million people each year. This tumor is most commonly detected in

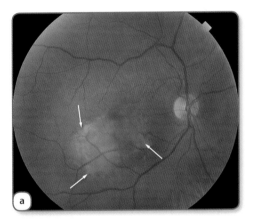
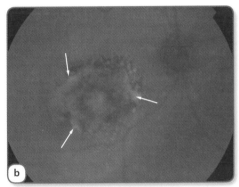

**Figure 61.4** Fundus autofluorescence (FAF) features of choroidal melanoma. (a) Fundus photograph of a choroidal melanoma with significant overlying lipofuscin (arrows). (b) Corresponding FAF image demonstrates hyperautofluorescence of the lipofuscin (arrows).

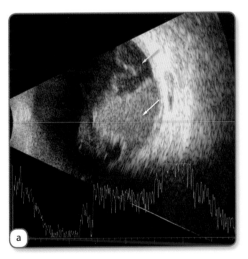
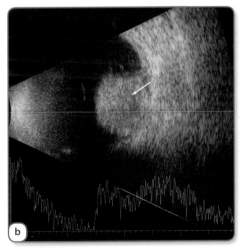

**Figure 61.5** Ultrasound features of choroidal melanoma. (a) A- and B-scan ultrasound of a choroidal melanoma demonstrating a classic mushroom or dome shape (white arrow) with associated serous retinal detachment (yellow arrow). (b) A- and B-scan ultrasound of a choroidal melanoma demonstrating characteristic dome shape, low-to-medium internal reflectivity, internal acoustic dampening, and excavation of the involved choroid.

the sixth decade of life and becomes more incident with increasing age; however, even young children can be affected. Choroidal melanoma is more common in lightly pigmented individuals.

## Symptoms and clinical findings

Associated serous retinal detachments and cystoid macular edema can cause decreased visual acuity and visual field deficits although smaller tumors may not cause any symptoms. Following treatment, visual loss can also occur as a result of radiation retinopathy and/or optic neuropathy.

The clinical appearance of a choroidal melanoma can be variable (**Figure 61.1**) but typically features a darkly pigmented, subretinal tumor that is dome-shaped and elevated, which enlarges without treatment (see Box). Associated clinical findings include the presence of surface lipofuscin (orange pigment) and overlying and adjacent serous subretinal fluid.

## Treatment/prognosis/follow-up

Choroidal melanoma is a malignant tumor with an overall mortality rate of approximately 50% over 10 years. The size of the tumor correlates with risk of metastasis and mortality with each 2 mm of tumor height beyond 8 mm corresponding to a worsening prognosis (**Table 61.1**). The decision and type of treatment should be made after careful consideration of all available clinical information. Small tumors can be observed closely with careful monitoring and serial photographs without any significant increased risk of metastasis. Most medium and large tumors are treated with radiation that can be applied

---

### Characteristic clinical features of choroidal melanoma

Size >5–10 mm diameter and >2 mm height
Associated serous retinal detachment
Proximity close to optic nerve
Overlying lipofuscin
Symptomatic
Enlargement over time

---

### Table 61.1 Choroidal melanoma size and risk of death from metastasis*

| Tumor size | Mortality rate at 5 years |
|---|---|
| Small (<10 mm diameter and <2–3 mm height) | <1% |
| Medium (<15 mm diameter and <5 mm height) | 37% |
| Large (>15 mm diameter and >5 mm height) | 57% |

*Shammas et al. (1977).

via numerous methods (plaque brachytherapy, charged particle radiation, gamma knife). Enucleation is reserved for very large tumors. Other additional treatment modalities that may be implored include transpupillary thermotherapy and laser photocoagulation, usually reserved as supplemental treatment in combination with radiation. Treatment serves to reduce the risk of metastasis and reduce mortality. Visual outcomes are often guarded due to effects from the tumor itself and radiation retinopathy. Metastases to the liver are most common and to the lung are second-most common. Metastatic workup prior to treatment is indicated and then annual surveillance is generally advisable, directed at the liver and lungs.

# Further reading

Shammas HF, Blodi FC. Prognostic factors in choroidal and ciliary body melanomas. Arch Ophthalmol 1977; 95:63–9.

# 62     Choroidal hemangioma

## How to approach a patient with a reddish-colored subretinal lesion

| Identify the primary pathologic clinical finding(s) | | |
|---|---|---|
| There is an orange/pink-colored, round subretinal lesion located within the macula (**Figure 62.1a**). | | |
| **Formulate a differential diagnosis** | | |
| Most likely | Less likely | Least likely |
| • Choroidal hemangioma | • Choroidal nevus, choroidal melanoma, choroidal hemorrhage, subretinal hemorrhage | • Choroidal osteoma, choroidal metastasis |
| **Query patient history** | | |
| • Is the patient experiencing any visual symptoms?<br>• Is there any history of systemic malignancy? | | |
| **Decide on ancillary diagnostic imaging** | | |
| Indocyanine green angiography (ICGA) and ultrasound imaging are the most useful ancillary tests in the evaluation of a suspected choroidal tumor. Fluorescein angiography and optical coherence tomography (OCT) may also provide useful additive information. | | |

## Ancillary diagnostic imaging interpretation

### Optical coherence tomography

OCT over the surface of a choroidal hemangioma can show associated subretinal fluid (**Figure 62.2**). In smaller tumors, shallow choroidal elevation caused by the tumor and subtle disruption of the choroid can be well visualized. OCT is most useful to monitor subretinal fluid or cystoid macular edema that may be present secondarily in the macula, particularly in response to treatment.

### Fluorescein angiography

Choroidal hemangiomas display diffuse hyperfluorescence of the entire tumor that develops early in a splotchy pattern and lasts throughout all phases of the angiogram, due to the inherent vascular nature of this tumor (**Figure 62.1b–d**). Small tumors may not be visualized with fluorescein angiography.

### Indocyanine green angiography

ICGA is the most useful ancillary diagnostic modality for smaller choroidal hemangiomas that are too small to image via ultrasound and in this situation can be the only confirmatory imaging modality. ICGA is also useful as an adjunct in larger tumors. There is characteristic bright

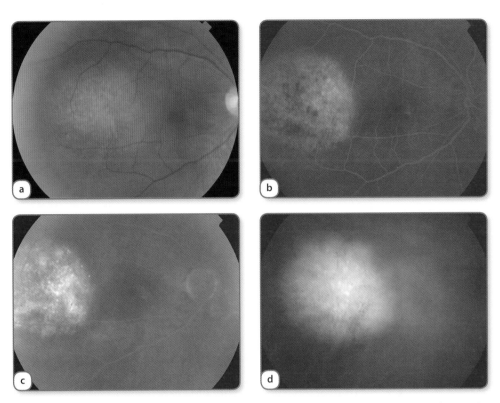

**Figure 62.1** Color photograph and fluorescein angiogram of a choroidal hemangioma (a–d). (a) Color photograph shows typical features of a circumscribed choroidal hemangioma in the macula. (b) Mid-phase angiogram shows mild diffuse hyperfluorescence of the lesion. (c, d) Later phase angiograms show increasing hyperfluorescence.

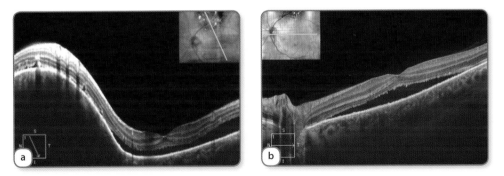

**Figure 62.2** Optical coherence tomography of a choroidal hemangioma (a, b). (a) There is a dome-shaped elevation underneath the retina (left side of image), which replaces the choroidal vasculature typically visible, and represents the choroidal hemangioma. There is shallow subretinal fluid overlying the tumor, which extends into the macula. (b) A typical line scan through the macula shows a more standard view of the subretinal fluid.

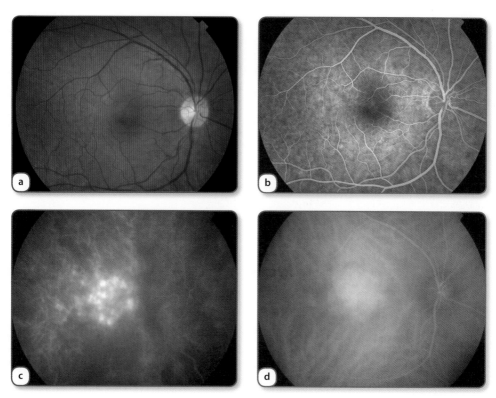

**Figure 62.3** Color photograph, fluorescein angiogram, and indocyanine green angiogram of a small choroidal hemangioma (a–d). (a) Color photograph shows a barely discernable, circumscribed choroidal hemangioma. (b) Fluorescein angiography does not reveal any prominent abnormality, except for faint staining. (c) Very early phase indocyanine green angiogram shows very prominent hyperfluorescence of the vasculature within the choroidal hemangioma, which is pathognomonic. (d) Later phase indocyanine green angiogram shows fading of the hyperfluorescence.

hyperfluorescence that begins in the very early phases of the angiogram corresponding to the inherent tumor vasculature (**Figure 62.3**), which eventually, and characteristically, fades very late (after 30+ minutes).

## Fundus autofluorescence

Fundus autofluorescence is not necessary but may provide supporting evidence to help confirm the diagnosis. Choroidal hemangiomas usually display no intrinsic autofluorescence or display hypoautofluorescence (**Figure 62.4**). In the minority of choroidal hemangiomas that have overlying orange pigment, hyperautofluorescence can be seen in these areas.

## Ultrasound

A- and B-scan ultrasound is one of the most important ancillary imaging modalities to confirm the diagnosis of choroidal hemangioma. A-scan ultrasound shows high internal acoustic reflectivity of the tumor (**Figure 62.5a**). B-scan ultrasound is used to measure the basal

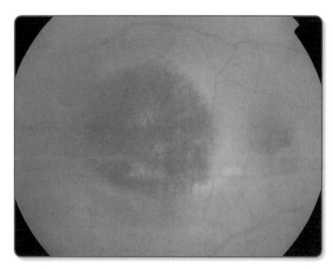

**Figure 62.4** Fundus autofluorescence of a choroidal hemangioma (corresponding to Figure 62.1). There is generalized hypoautofluorescence in the region of the tumor.

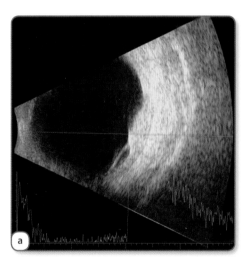

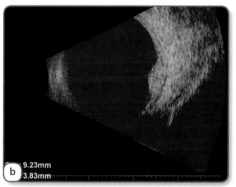

**Figure 62.5** A- and B-scan ultrasound of a choroidal hemangioma. (a) A-scan ultrasound demonstrates typical high internal reflectivity. (b) B-scan ultrasound demonstrates localized thickening of the choroid in the region of the tumor without any choroidal excavation (seen in choroidal melanoma, see Chapter 61).

dimensions and height of the tumor (**Figure 62.5b**) and typically shows a smooth, dome-shaped elevation of the choroid.

# Final diagnosis: circumscribed choroidal hemangioma

## Epidemiology/etiology

Choroidal hemangiomas are an uncommon benign vascular hamartoma involving the choroid. There are two forms of choroidal hemangioma: circumscribed and diffuse. The circumscribed form is more common and occurs as an isolated finding, while the diffuse form is typically seen in association with certain systemic syndromes such as Sturge–Weber syndrome.

## Symptoms and clinical findings

Circumscribed choroidal hemangiomas commonly cause no symptoms, although a hyperopic shift may be present if the tumor is located under the macula. In the presence of secondary effects of the tumor such as overlying or adjacent serous retinal detachments and/or cystoid macular edema, patients may experience decreased visual acuity or metamorphopsia.

Circumscribed choroidal hemangiomas are orange to red-colored choroidal tumors that are round with ill-defined edges and typically located in the posterior pole of the fundus. They are typically mildly elevated (<4 mm in thickness). Diffuse choroidal hemangiomas may involve most or all of the entire choroid causing a diffuse reddish thickening and discoloration.

## Treatment/prognosis/follow-up

Asmyptomatic tumors may be observed as the tumor itself is benign. If there are associated secondary effects in the retina affecting the vision (such as subretinal fluid or cystoid macular edema), then treatment may be necessary. Traditional treatment options include laser photocoagulation, photodynamic therapy, radiation therapy, and transpupillary thermotherapy. Laser photocoagulation can be applied lightly to the surface of a circumscribed choroidal hemangioma to decrease subretinal fluid secretion (**Figure 62.6**). Photodynamic therapy is applied using a spot size equivalent to the diameter of the circumscribed choroidal hemangioma and may be successful in reducing associated serous retinal detachments. External radiation is

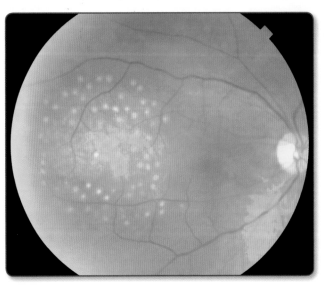

**Figure 62.6**  Color photograph of choroidal hemangioma immediately following treatment with laser photocoagulation.

typically reserved for larger tumors or those recalcitrant to alternative modes of treatment. More recently, anti-VEGF in the form of intravitreal bevacizumab has been use as monotherapy or in combination with traditional treatment modalities in the management of symptomatic circumscribed choroidal hemangiomas.

# Further reading

Kwon HJ, Kim M, Lee CS, Lee SC. Treatment of serous macular detachment associated with circumscribed choroidal hemangioma. Am J Ophthalmol 2012; 154:137–45.

Mandal S, Naithani P, Venkatesh P, Garg S. Intravitreal bevacizumab (Avastin) for circumscribed choroidal hemangioma. Indian J Ophthalmol 2011; 59:248–51.

## How to approach a patient with a saccular, vascular cluster overlying the retina

| Identify the primary pathologic clinical finding(s) | | |
|---|---|---|
| There is a localized, saccular vascular anomaly that resembles a cluster of grapes located on the surface of the retina (**Figure 63.1**). | | |
| Formulate a differential diagnosis | | |
| **Most likely** | **Less likely** | **Least likely** |
| • Retinal cavernous hemangioma | • Retinal capillary hemangioma, coats disease | • Neovascularization of the retina |
| Query patient history | | |
| • Has this lesion been noted before?<br>• Are there any problems with vision?<br>• Is there a history of von Hippel–Lindau syndrome? | | |
| Decide on ancillary diagnostic imaging | | |
| Clinical examination reveals characteristic features. Fluorescein angiography (FA) can be confirmatory. | | |

## Ancillary diagnostic imaging interpretation

### Fluorescein angiography

There are characteristic features on FA, which help to distinguish retinal cavernous hemangiomas from other similar entities (**Figure 63.2b**). The cavernous vascular abnormalities exhibit delayed filling with fluorescein during the venous phase. There is reverse pooling of fluorescein superiorly due to staining of plasma because of red blood cells settling dependently. Characteristically, there is no associated hyperfluorescence or leakage of fluorescein and no feeder vessels (distinguishes from retinal capillary hemangiomas).

### Color photography

Color photographs are useful only to document the current appearance of this lesion.

## Final diagnosis: retinal cavernous hemangioma

### Epidemiology/etiology

Retinal cavernous hemangiomas are believed to be congenital vascular hamartomas, which are typically unilateral and stable in size over time. They are typically an isolated finding, although rare reports have documented syndromic patients with cavernous hemangiomas in other organ systems (skin and central nervous system).

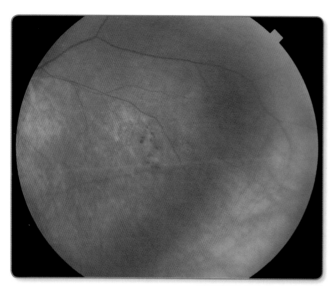

**Figure 63.1** Color photograph of a retinal cavernous hemangioma showing characteristic appearance of a smaller lesion.

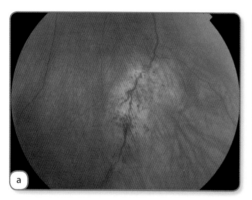

a

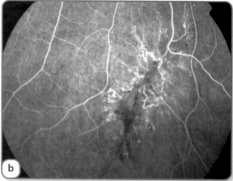

b

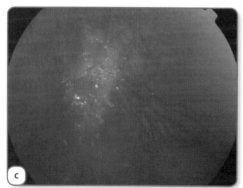

c

**Figure 63.2** Color photograph (a) and corresponding fluorescein angiogram (b, c) of a retinal cavernous hemangioma. Fluorescein angiogram shows delayed filling of the cavernous vascular lesions in the venous phase (b) followed by bright staining of the plasma component within the vascular lesions in the later phase angiogram (c).

## Symptoms and clinical findings

Most patients are asymptomatic although symptoms can be present depending on the location of the lesion and any associated secondary effects such as epiretinal membrane or vitreous hemorrhage. Retinal cavernous hemangiomas have a very characteristic clinical appearance due to a dense cluster of saccular aneurysms, which resemble a cluster of grapes (**Figure 63.1**). The size and location of the lesions can be highly variable. There is typically one localized cluster of aneurysms although multifocal lesions are possible. Associated subretinal fluid, exudates, or feeder vessels (features of retinal capillary hemangiomas) are not seen. Overlying preretinal fibrosis may be present.

## Treatment/prognosis/follow-up

Making the correct diagnosis is critical as no treatment or further workup is generally indicated for this benign lesion. Depending on any associated features (and severity), such as epiretinal membrane, directed treatment may be necessary.

## How to approach a patient with vascular lesion in the retina

| Identify the primary pathologic clinical finding(s) | | |
|---|---|---|
| There is one or more spherical, red-colored vascular lesion(s) located on the surface of the retina and/or optic nerve associated with dilated and tortuous retinal vessels (**Figure 64.1a**). | | |
| Formulate a differential diagnosis | | |
| **Most likely** | **Less likely** | **Least likely** |
| • Retinal capillary hemangioma | • Coats disease, vasoproliferative tumor, retinal macroaneurysm | • Familial exudative vitreoretinopathy, exudative retinal detachment, retinal astrocytoma |
| Query patient history | | |
| • Does the patient have any known personal or family history of von Hippel–Lindau syndrome?<br>• Does the patient have any other systemic problems such as kidney problems, high blood pressure, or headaches?<br>• Are there findings in one eye or both eyes? | | |
| Decide on ancillary diagnostic imaging | | |
| The diagnosis is usually made initially based on clinical examination, though ancillary diagnostic testing can be helpful for confirmation. Fundus photographs are useful to document the current lesion appearance and to help document any changes in size over time. Fluorescein angiography (FA) is the most useful ancillary diagnostic test to confirm the diagnosis of a retinal capillary hemangioma. Optical coherence tomography (OCT) can provide useful information about the lesion if a scan can be taken through the lesion itself. Additionally, OCT is useful to monitor secondary effects in the macula such as subretinal fluid or macular edema, particularly in making a decision for treatment or to guide response following treatment. | | |

## Ancillary diagnostic imaging interpretation

### Optical coherence tomography

OCT is helpful to identify any associated intra- or subretinal fluid, which may be affecting the macula (**Figure 64.2**). Following treatment, OCT is critical to detect any treatment response in such patients.

### Fluorescein angiography

FA shows a characteristic leakage pattern and is particularly helpful to identify the presence of feeder vessels (**Figure 64.3**), which may be subtle.

### Color photography

Color photographs are useful to document changes in lesion size and any associated exudative retinal detachment that may be present (**Figure 64.1b**). Widefield imaging modalities or montage photographs are optimal for detection and monitoring of peripheral lesions.

## Final diagnosis: retinal capillary hemangioma (or hemangioblastoma)

### Epidemiology/etiology

Retinal capillary hemangiomas (or hemangioblastomas) are benign hamartomatous, vascular tumors, which can become visually

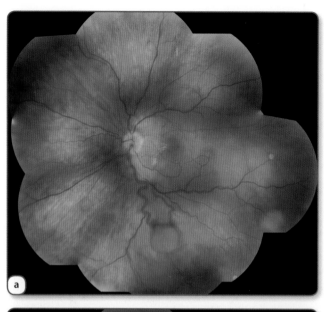

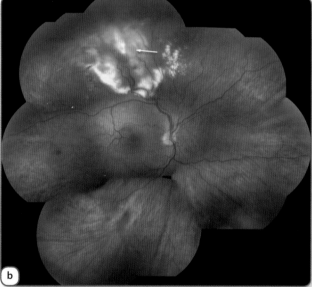

**Figure 64.1** Color photographs of retinal capillary hemangiomas. (a) A characteristic retinal capillary hemangioma is shown with typical dilated and tortuous feeding/draining vessels. There is mild exudation into the nasal macula. (b) A characteristic retinal capillary hemangioma (arrow) is present superiorly along with a surrounding exudative retinal detachment, which is outside of the macula.

significant via secondary structural effects on the neighboring retinal tissue. An isolated retinal capillary hemangioma is termed von Hippel disease, whereas if multiple or bilateral retinal capillary hemangiomas are seen in association with various other systemic hemangioblastomas, the term von Hippel–Lindau syndrome is used. Von Hippel–Lindau syndrome is a rare autosomal dominant disease, caused by a defect on chromosome 3 affecting the *VHL* gene. Genetic testing is available to confirm the diagnosis. Patients with the syndrome are at risk for a

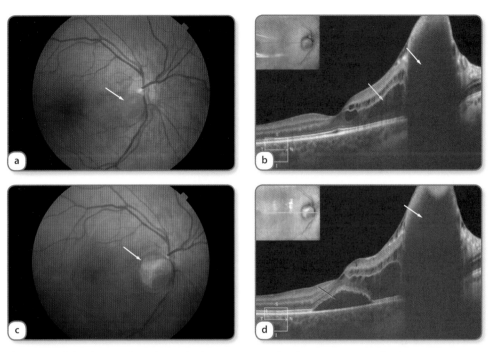

**Figure 64.2** Color photographs and optical coherence tomography of an optic nerve capillary hemangioma in a patient with von Hippel–Lindau syndrome. (a, b) An optic nerve capillary hemangioma (white arrows) and associated cystoid macular edema (yellow arrow) are illustrated. Note that typical feeder vessels are not present with optic nerve hemangiomas. (c, d) Nine months later, the capillary hemangioma (white arrows) has enlarged in size with development of subretinal fluid (red arrow), which adversely affected visual acuity.

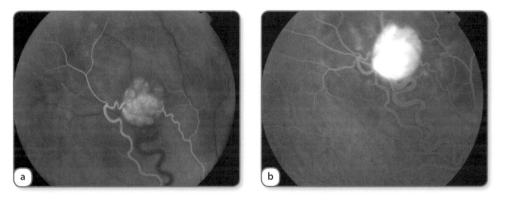

**Figure 64.3** Fluorescein angiography of a retinal capillary hemangioma. There is characteristic early hyperfluorescence of the lesion (a) followed by continued leakage in later frames (b).

variety of systemic malignancies and cysts involving the brain, kidneys, adrenal glands, pancreas, and epididymis.

## Symptoms and clinical findings

Smaller tumors may only appear as a small red area in the retina, whereas larger tumors have a more characteristic spherical or oblong angiomatous appearance. Unless very small, typical feeder and draining retinal vessels that are dilated and tortuous should be present. Lesions may be isolated and unilateral in sporadic cases (Figure 64.1) or may be multifocal and bilateral in syndromic cases (**Figure 64.4**). Rarely, hemangiomas may involve the optic nerve head instead of, or in addition to the retina (Figure 64.2).

Symptoms can be caused by associated sub- and intraretinal exudation, which may involve the macula (Figure 64.2). Secondary epiretinal membranes and, rarely, tractional retinal detachments may also be present. Symptoms may include decreased visual acuity, metamorphopsia, or a decreased visual field.

## Treatment/prognosis/follow-up

If von Hippel–Lindau syndrome is suspected, further systemic evaluation with a multidiscipline team should be coordinated by the patients' primary care provider, which should be focused on workup for pheochromocytoma, renal cell carcinoma, cerebellar hemangioblastomas, islet cell tumors, and epididymal cysts.

Retinal capillary hemangiomas are best identified and treated early, when small and not causing secondary complications, as the majority of these tumors progressively grow over time. Once complications develop, treatment response declines and visual prognosis is guarded. Treatment options for retinal capillary hemangiomas include direct laser photocoagulation, cryotherapy, external radiation, photodynamic therapy, and observation. Intravitreal anti-VEGF therapy has been attempted but appears to have minimal if any benefit. Capillary hemangiomas involving the optic nerve are usually observed initially

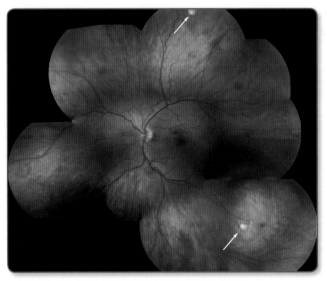

**Figure 64.4** Color photographs of multifocal retinal capillary hemangiomas (fellow eye corresponds to Figure 64.1b). In a patient with von Hippel–Lindau syndrome, multiple retinal capillary hemangiomas are present in the same eye (arrows).

until causing symptoms, due to the high risk of adverse visual effects from the treatment in this location.

Patients with retinal capillary hemangiomas should be followed at regular intervals to help detect any significant clinical changes, which may impact vision. Family members of patients with von Hippel–Lindau syndrome should be appropriately counseled and screened for disease.

# Further reading

Papastefanou VP, Pilli S, Stinghe A, Lotery AJ, Cohen VM. Photodynamic therapy for retinal capillary hemangioma. Eye (Lond) 2013; 27:438–42.

# Combined hamartoma of the retina and retinal pigment epithelium

## How to approach a patient with a pigmented fundus lesion involving the retina and overlying retinal vasculature

| Identify the primary pathologic clinical finding(s) | | |
|---|---|---|
| There is a pigmented lesion with irregular edges located in the macula adjacent to the optic nerve that appears to involve the full thickness of the retina with overlying fibrous membranes and focal contracture of the retinal vasculature (**Figure 65.1**). | | |
| **Formulate a differential diagnosis** | | |
| **Most likely** | **Less likely** | **Least likely** |
| • Combined hamartoma of the retina and retinal pigment epithelium | • Choroidal melanoma, choroidal nevus, congenital hypertrophy of the retinal pigment epithelium, melanocytoma | • Epiretinal membrane, retinoblastoma, hemangioma, astrocytoma |
| **Query patient history** | | |
| • If this is in a child, is there any associated strabismus or ocular misalignment?<br>• If this is an adult, has the lesion been noted before?<br>• Is the lesion changing in size?<br>• Are there any associated visual symptoms? | | |
| **Decide on ancillary diagnostic imaging** | | |
| This condition has a characteristic clinical appearance but diagnostic testing can be very helpful to exclude some of the more serious conditions being considered in the differential diagnosis. Useful diagnostic testing include optical coherence tomography (OCT), fluorescein angiography (FA), and B-scan ultrasound in certain cases. | | |

## Ancillary diagnostic imaging interpretation

### Optical coherence tomography

Typical OCT features include a dense overlying epiretinal membrane that has a corrugated appearance. The underlying retinal layers and retinal pigment epithelium (RPE) are contracted and disorganized with loss of clear distinctions between layers (**Figure 65.2a**). The overlying fibrous membranes display bright hyper-reflectivity. Cystic edema may be seen on the edges (**Figure 65.2b**).

### Fluorescein angiography

This lesion displays characteristic features on FA, which help confirm the diagnosis (**Figure 65.3**). The superficial portion of the lesion encompasses abnormal vasculature, which creates a corkscrew-like, tortuous matrix that is best visualized on FA. These vessels display significant late hyperfluorescence. There is blockage from the deeper pigmented portions of the lesion and also may be areas that in a serpiginous fashion.

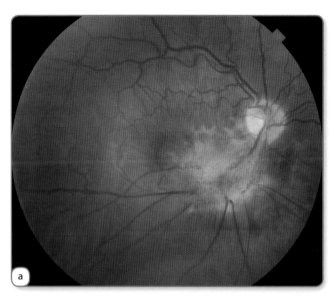

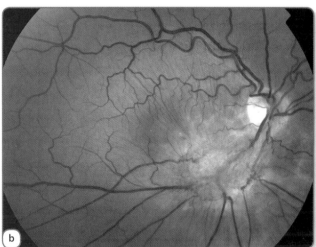

**Figure 65.1** Color (a) and red-free (b) photograph of combined hamartoma of the retina and RPE. A typical combined hamartoma with macular involvement is shown. (a) The lesion has grayish coloration and involves the retina and overlying vasculature while obscuring the underlying RPE. There is a characteristic overlying preretinal fibrous membrane. (b) Some features are better visualized on red-free images.

# Final diagnosis: combined hamartoma of the retina and RPE

## Epidemiology/etiology

Combined hamartoma of the retina and RPE most likely arises as a developmental aberration, which encompasses the RPE, retina, and overlying vasculature, which are all involved to varying degrees. It is usually first recognized in childhood, although presentation in adulthood is possible in milder cases, particularly if the macula is spared. Rarely, this condition may be associated with systemic conditions such as neurofibromatosis.

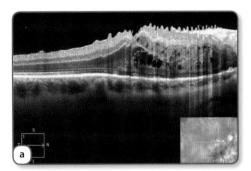
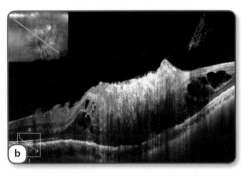

**Figure 65.2** Optical coherence tomography of combined hamartoma of the retina and RPE (corresponding to Figure 65.1). (a) A horizontal line scan through the macula shows a clear distinction between uninvolved retina (temporal) and involved retina (nasal). The involved portion displays characteristic optical coherence tomography features including a corrugated epiretinal membrane with loss of retinal layer/RPE organization and associated cystic intraretinal spaces. (b) Diagonal line scan through the lesion illustrates the prominent preretinal fibrous membrane that is hyper-reflective, which creates a shadowing artifact making underlying structures poorly visualized. There are intraretinal cystic changes on the edge of the lesion.

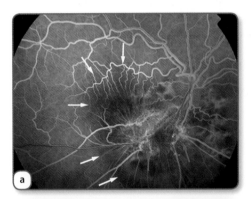
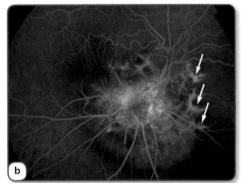

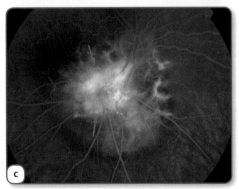

**Figure 65.3** Fluorescein angiogram of combined hamartoma of the retina and RPE. (a) Early phase angiogram illustrates widespread blockage of background fluorescence (white arrows) and the abnormal superficial, fine, corkscrew-like vascular meshwork (red arrows). (b) Mid-phase angiogram further highlights the superficial vascular anomalies (red arrows) and reveals serpiginous areas of deep staining (white arrows). (c) Late phase angiogram shows hyperfluorescence of the superficial vessels (red arrows).

## Symptoms and clinical findings

Symptoms depend on the age, presentation, and severity but may include decreased visual acuity, strabismus, and metamorphopsia. Visual acuity can range from normal to worse than 20/200. Mild cases may be asymptomatic and diagnosed incidentally. This entity is a rare, benign, hamartomatous tumor that has a dark gray coloration, is slightly elevated, has feathery edges, may involve the macula or periphery, has overlying fibrotic membranes that distort nearby vasculature, and is typically unilateral.

## Treatment/prognosis/follow-up

It is important to differentiate this lesion from others listed in the differential diagnosis (particularly choroidal melanoma and retinoblastoma) because combined hamartoma of the retina and RPE is a benign condition and confusion for certain other conditions may lead to unnecessarily invasive treatment. Over time, this condition is slowly progressive and, generally, no treatment is indicated. Surgical removal of associated epiretinal membranes via vitrectomy with membrane peeling may be considered in certain cases, but carries a guarded prognosis for improvement of vision.

# Further reading

Shields CL, Thangappan A, Hartzell K, et al. Combined hamartoma of the retina and retinal pigment epithelium in 77 consecutive patients visual outcome based on macular versus extramacular tumor location. Ophthalmology 2008; 115:2246.

# How to approach a pediatric patient with leukocoria

| Identify the primary pathologic clinical finding(s) | | |
|---|---|---|
| There is leukocoria of the right eye (**Figure 66.1a**). Behind a clear lens, an elevated, chalky-white mass is visible (**Figure 66.1b**) | | |
| **Formulate a differential diagnosis** | | |
| **Most likely** | **Less likely** | **Least likely** |
| • Retinoblastoma | • Persistent fetal vasculature, retinal astrocytic hamartoma, Coats' disease, toxocariasis | • Familial exudative vitreoretinopathy, retinopathy of prematurity, retinal detachment, endophthalmitis, cataract, combined hamartoma, coloboma |
| **Query patient history** | | |
| • Is there any family history of retinoblastoma?<br>• Is there any family history of other malignancies?<br>• Have there been any other health concerns during pregnancy or infancy?<br>• Does the affected eye ever turn in or out unexpectedly? | | |
| **Decide on ancillary diagnostic imaging** | | |
| An examination under anesthesia with fundus photography, fluorescein angiography, and ultrasonography are important in the evaluation of this patient, although the clinical appearance alone is typically sufficient to make the diagnosis. CT imaging is usually avoided to prevent unnecessary radiation exposure that may increase the likelihood for a secondary malignancy. MRI is preferred for staging to assess the extent of any invasion through the optic nerve into the orbit and/or brain. Pathologic evaluation of enucleated specimens can confirm the diagnosis. Needle biopsy is not recommended due to the risk of seeding outside the eye. | | |

# Ancillary diagnostic imaging interpretation

## Fluorescein angiography

A fine capillary network is often present on the surface of retinoblastoma tumors, which are more easily visualized on angiography and show hyperfluorescence (**Figure 66.2**).

## Ultrasonography

Ultrasound can be used to detect the presence of intratumor calcifications, which show increased reflectivity with posterior shadowing.

## Histopathology

Characteristic histologic features of retinoblastoma include abundant hyperchromatic nuclei with minimal cytoplasm and high mitotic activity (**Figure 66.3**). Tumor cells aggregate near blood vessels, which they are heavily depend on for growth, which results in a characteristic pattern of necrosis that starts about 100 µm away from blood vessels. Flexner–Wintersteiner rosettes and Homer Wright rosettes may be identified, the former being most specific to retinoblastoma.

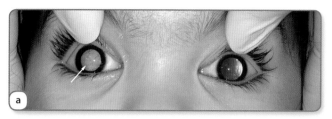
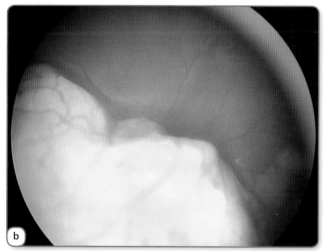

**Figure 66.1** Typical presentation of retinoblastoma. (a) A classic example of leukocoria is shown (arrow), whereas the fellow eye has an intact red reflex. (b) Corresponding Retcam photograph of the fundus reveals a large intraretinal tumor that obliterates normal retinal landmarks.

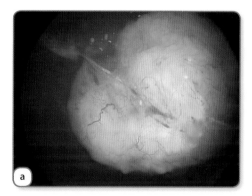
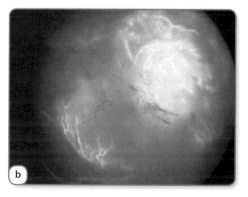

**Figure 66.2** Fluorescein angiography in retinoblastoma. Color photograph (a) with corresponding fluorescein angiogram (b) shows prominent fine vessels along the surface of the tumor, which show hyperfluorescence.

# Final diagnosis: retinoblastoma

## Epidemiology/etiology

Retinoblastoma is the most common intraocular malignancy in children occurring in about 1 in 15,000 births, typically diagnosed before 3 years of age. The diagnosis is critical to keep in mind in the differential diagnosis of leukocoria due to its potentially serious systemic consequences. This malignant tumor is thought to arise

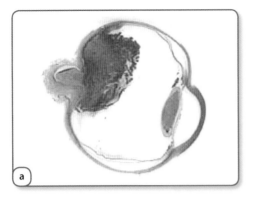

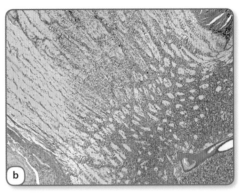

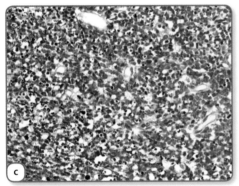

**Figure 66.3** Histopathology in retinoblastoma (corresponding to Figure 66.2). Characteristic histopathologic features of retinoblastoma are shown with increasing magnification from a–c. (a) A pupil-optic nerve globe section is shown with the tumor occupying the posterior extent of the eye. A prominence of dark-colored staining is present in the tumor, reflecting the high amount of nuclear material and lack of cytoplasm. (b) Optic nerve invasion is present. (c) Higher magnification view of the tumor cells.

from retinal photoreceptor cells. The genetics of retinoblastoma are well understood with defects in the *RB1* gene (a tumor suppressor gene), located on chromosome 13, implicated in the pathogenesis. Inactivation of both copies of this gene results in development of retinoblastoma. The majority of cases are unilateral and sporadic, although offspring of an affected patient with a germline mutation and bilateral disease have a 45% chance of being affected.

Histopathologic features of retinoblastoma include nuclei with an extremely high mitotic rate that appear dark due to increased amounts of chromatin (**Figure 66.3a–c**).

## Symptoms and clinical findings

The most common presenting sign is leukocoria (see Box), though other common signs and symptoms include strabismus, intraocular inflammation, pseudo-hypopyon, hyphema, decreased vision, proptosis, and pain.

Large retinoblastoma tumors have a characteristic chalky-white clinical appearance (**Figures 66.1** and **66.2**). The tumor may be endophytic (growing on the retinal surface) or exophytic (growing under the retina) and intratumor calcification is a characteristic feature Satellite retinal lesions and vitreous seeding may be present due to shedding of viable cells or multifocality. Tumors identified early may

## Differential diagnosis of leukocoria in a child

Retinoblastoma
Persistent fetal vasculature
Retinal astrocytic hamartoma
Coats disease
Toxocariasis
Familial exudative vitreoretinopathy
Retinopathy of prematurity
Retinal detachment
Endophthalmitis
Cataract
Combined hamartoma
Coloboma

be much smaller and appear semitranslucent or gray with prominent retinal vessels. Eyes with retinoblastoma are typically normal in size, a feature that is helpful in differentiation from persistent fetal vasculature where eyes are typically nanophthalmic.

## Treatment/prognosis/follow-up

A thorough examination under anesthesia is the first step in evaluation of a child with suspected retinoblastoma. If the tumor is confined to the globe, prognosis for survival is excellent with a >95% survival rate. If the tumor has invaded out of the globe (usually via the optic nerve or the choroid) and/or metastasized, survival rates drop to 50% or less. Treatment priority is two tiered with survival first and vision-preservation second. There are a variety of treatment options that are individually tailored depending on size and location of tumor involvement, bilaterality, and whether extraocular extension is present. Treatment modalities include enucleation (reserved for larger tumors with poor visual prognosis), external radiation, cryotherapy (reserved for small tumors), laser photocoagulation (reserved for small tumors), and systemic and intra-arterial tumor chemotherapy

Genetic counseling to family members is important, particularly in bilateral cases where a germline mutation is suspected. Secondary malignancies are common later in life in patients with germline mutations, who survive to adulthood. These secondary malignancies include pinealomas, bone and soft tissue sarcomas, and cutaneous melanomas.

# Further reading

Shields CL, Shields JA. Diagnosis and management of retinoblastoma. Cancer Control 2004; 11:317–27.
Shields CL, Shields JA. Basic understanding of current classification and management of retinoblastoma. Curr Opin Ophthalmol 2006; 17:228–34.

## How to approach a patient with an unexpected choroidal mass

| Identify the primary pathologic clinical finding(s) | | |
|---|---|---|
| There is a yellow-colored, dome-shaped subretinal lesion located in the posterior pole (**Figure 67.1**). | | |
| **Formulate a differential diagnosis** | | |
| **Most likely** | **Less likely** | **Least likely** |
| • Choroidal metastasis | • Amelanotic choroidal melanoma or nevus, choroidal hemangioma, posterior scleritis | • Choroidal osteoma, Vogt–Koyanagi–Harada syndrome, disciform scar, rhegmatogenous retinal detachment, endogenous endophthalmitis |
| **Query patient history** | | |
| • Is there any known history of systemic malignancy?<br>• Is the patient experiencing any fevers, chills, night sweats, weight loss, unusual lumps or rashes, fatigue, or general malaise?<br>• Is the eye painful?<br>• Is the patient a current or former smoker? | | |
| **Decide on ancillary diagnostic imaging** | | |
| Clinical examination in the context of a known systemic malignancy is typically enough to make the diagnosis. In cases where there is diagnostic uncertainty or no known primary malignancy, fluorescein angiography and ultrasonography can be informative. In very small tumors, optical coherence tomography may be more sensitive than traditional ultrasound. Color, red free, and fundus autofluorescence (FAF) images can provide additional information toward confirming a diagnosis. Biopsy is reserved for particularly unusual cases. | | |

## Ancillary diagnostic imaging interpretation

### Fluorescein angiography

The circulation and fluorescence pattern are useful to differentiate metastatic choroidal tumors from primary choroidal melanomas (which often have a double circulation) and other intraocular tumors. In choroidal metastasis, there is typically early blockage followed by late leakage over the area of the tumor and there is more likely to be multiple pinpoint areas of leakage. The early areas of blockage are useful to define the tumor margins (**Figure 67.2**).

### Fundus autofluorescence

Choroidal metastatic tumors can display a variety of findings on FAF. Pigmented areas on the tumor surface are typically hyperautofluorescent, which form a mottled pattern along with areas of hypo autofluorescence. The pattern created by the mix of hypo- and hyperautofluorescence can help delineate the tumor margins (**Figure 67.3**).

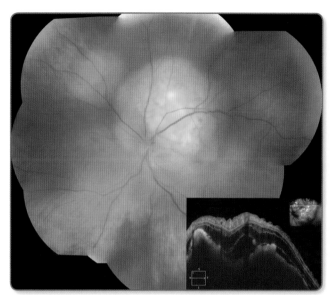

**Figure 67.1** Color photograph and corresponding optical coherence tomography of a metastatic choroidal tumor (presumed pulmonary). There is a large, elevated amelanotic subretinal lesion located in the choroid. Optical coherence tomography line scan through the center of the tumor is shown (inset).

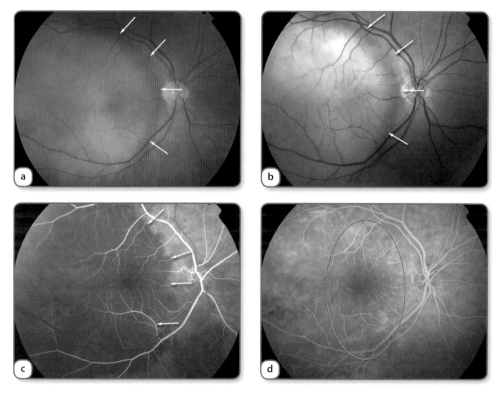

**Figure 67.2** Fluorescein angiography of a metastatic choroidal tumor. (a) Color photograph and (b) red-free photograph are shown corresponding to the fluorescein angiogram. (c) Early phase angiogram shows hypofluorescence due to blockage from the tumor, which helps delineate the tumor margins (arrows). (d) Later phase angiogram shows mottled diffuse hyperfluorescence of the tumor in addition to multiple pinpoint areas of leakage (within red circle), which are characteristic of a metastatic carcinoma.

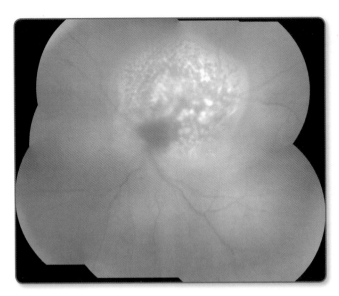

**Figure 67.3** Fundus autofluorescence of a metastatic choroidal tumor (corresponding to Figure 67.1). There is splotchy hyperautofluorescence of pigment changes overlying the tumor alternating with background hypoautofluorescence. The margins of the tumor are well illustrated.

## Red-free photography

Red-free photographs can help demonstrate tumor margins (**Figure 67.2b**).

## Color photography

Color photographs can help to detect any changes in size of metastatic tumors, which can grow quickly (**Figure 67.4**).

## Ultrasonography

A- and B-scan ultrasound shows characteristic features in metastatic choroidal tumors (**Figure 67.5**). A scan will typically show medium-to-high internal reflectivity. B scan is useful to measure tumor dimensions and detect the presence of any associated serous retinal detachment.

# Final diagnosis: choroidal metastasis

## Epidemiology/etiology

Metastatic disease involving the eye is rare, although this is the most common etiology of intraocular malignancies. The uveal tract, particularly the choroid, is the most common ocular location of involvement. Various types of solid tumors may metastasize to the eye but the four most common are carcinomas originating from the breast, lungs, from an unknown origin, and the gastrointestinal tract (see Box overleaf). Disease is typically unilateral although bilaterality is far more common in metastatic breast carcinoma than with other metastatic tumors.

Knowledge of a known, currently active or previously treated, systemic malignancy is present in about two thirds of suspected metastatic choroidal tumors (more commonly if the primary is breast

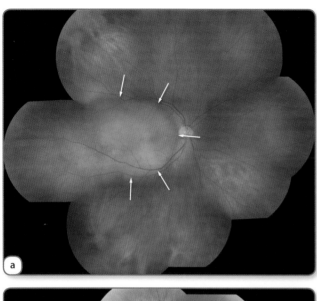

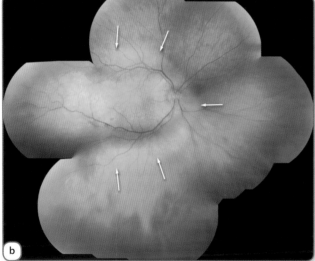

**Figure 67.4** Color photos of a metastatic choroidal tumor showing significant enlargement over an 8-week period: (a) baseline and (b) 8 weeks later. The edges of the tumor are highlighted by arrows.

carcinoma and less commonly if the primary is lung carcinoma). Not infrequently, however, a suspected choroidal metastasis is identified in the absence of any known systemic primary malignancy. In this situation, targeted workup to look for the most common systemic malignancies should be initiated with lung carcinoma being most likely. Despite careful investigation, a primary tumor is not identified in 50% of such cases.

## Symptoms and clinical findings

Patients with metastatic choroidal tumors are usually symptomatic with decreased visual acuity, photopsias, floaters, or pain. The minority of patients may have no symptoms.

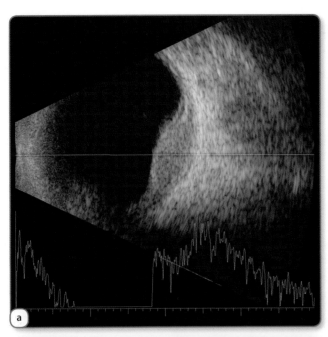

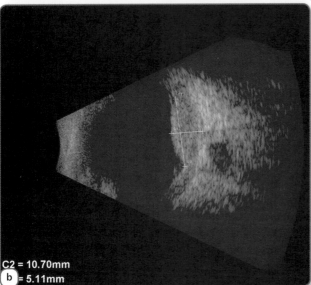

**Figure 67.5** A- and B-scan ultrasound of a metastatic choroidal tumor. (a) A-scan ultrasound shows medium internal reflectivity. (b) B-scan ultrasound illustrates how tumor dimensions are measured.

Metastatic choroidal carcinomas are usually amelanotic or yellowish in color and can be singular or multifocal. They are typically round, elevated tumors (Figure 67.1) with surrounding subretinal fluid but may take on a plate-like appearance (Figure 67.2).

## Treatment/prognosis/follow-up

Treatment for metastatic choroidal tumors usually takes on a palliative approach with the goals of visual preservation and comfort. Systemic

---

## Most common source for uveal metastatic tumors after a careful systemic investigation

Breast (47%)
Lung (21%)
Unknown (17%)
Gastrointestinal (2%)
Kidney (2%)
Modified from Shields et al. (1997).

---

chemotherapy directed at the primary malignancy is often sufficient to achieve a beneficial effect on the choroidal tumor. In cases where systemic therapy fails to achieve the desired effect on the ocular tumor, directed local therapy may be considered. The decision to initiate local treatment should consider the overall well-being of the patient, the significance of vision loss or threat to vision loss, laterality, and status of the fellow eye. Modalities for local therapy include external radiation, intravitreal injection, cryotherapy, photodynamic therapy, and thermal laser therapy.

The presence of a metastatic tumor in the choroid is indicative of a grave prognosis, as this usually is associated with widespread systemic metastases.

## Reference

Shields CL, Shields JA, Gross NE, Schwartz GP, Lally SE. Survey of 520 eyes with uveal metastases. Ophthalmology 1997; 104:1265–76.

## Further reading

Chen CJ, McCoy AN, Brahmer J, Handa JT. Emerging treatments for choroidal metastases. Surv Ophthalmol 2011; 56:511–21.
Demirci H, Shields CL, Chao AN, Shields JA. Uveal metastasis from breast cancer in 264 patients. Am J Ophthalmol 2003; 136:264–71.
Shah SU, Mashayekhi A, Shields CL, et al. Uveal metastasis from lung cancer: clinical features, treatment, and outcome in 194 patients. Ophthalmology 2014; 121:352–7.

# Section 10

# Trauma

# How to approach a patient with a crescent-shaped defect in the macula following blunt trauma

| Identify the primary pathologic clinical finding(s) | | |
| --- | --- | --- |
| There is a well-circumscribed subretinal defect that is somewhat linear and oriented vertically in the temporal macula (Figure 69.1). | | |
| Formulate a differential diagnosis | | |
| Most likely | Less likely | Least likely |
| • Choroidal rupture | • Commotio retinae, sclopetaria | • Choroidal neovascular membrane |
| Query patient history | | |
| • How recent was the traumatic injury?<br>• What kind of traumatic injury occurred (i.e. blunt trauma)?<br>• Was there subretinal hemorrhage initially overlying the area of concern?<br>• Does the patient have any features suggestive of angioid streaks, high myopia, or age-related macular degeneration in the fellow eye? | | |
| Decide on ancillary diagnostic imaging | | |
| Optical coherence tomography (OCT) and fluorescein angiography (FA) can be used to confirm the presence of a suspected choroidal rupture site. Indocyanine green angiography can be used as an alternative to FA. Depending on the amount and degree of overlying hemorrhage, these ancillary diagnostic studies may need to be delayed a period of time after the initial injury to allow for clearing of the hemorrhage. | | |

## Ancillary diagnostic imaging interpretation

### Optical coherence tomography

OCT is only useful if a small amount or no overlying hemorrhage is present because significant hemorrhage will prevent adequate signal penetration. The appearance of a choroidal rupture site is characteristic on OCT (**Figure 69.2**) as focal areas of loss of the retinal pigment epithelium (RPE)/Bruch's membrane complex and inner choroid.

### Fluorescein angiography

FA is useful to identify the extent and location of a choroidal rupture site, as the margins are sharply visualized as bright staining (**Figure 69.3b**). This imaging modality is also limited by the amount and degree of any overlying hemorrhage present. FA is also useful to evaluate for the presence of any secondary choroidal neovascular membrane that may develop in the setting of a choroidal rupture.

## Final diagnosis: choroidal rupture

### Epidemiology/etiology

Choroidal ruptures occur as an indirect result of significant blunt ocular trauma. The forces of the injury cause compression of the globe

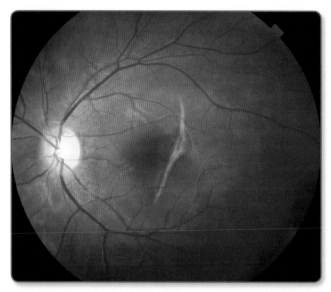

**Figure 69.1** Color photograph of choroidal rupture. Many months after the initial blunt traumatic injury, there is a choroidal rupture site visible in the temporal macula, which was initially obscured by overlying hemorrhage. The affected area spares the fovea and is slightly elevated and located below the retina.

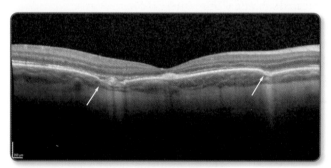

**Figure 69.2** Optical coherence tomography of choroidal rupture. Two focal defects in the retinal pigment epithelium (RPE)/Bruch's membrane complex are shown (arrows), which represent two separate choroidal rupture sites. There is reverse shadowing in both of these regions as a result of loss of the highly reflective RPE in these regions. Courtesy of Jeffrey Heier, MD.

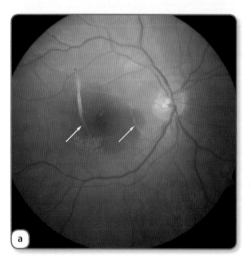

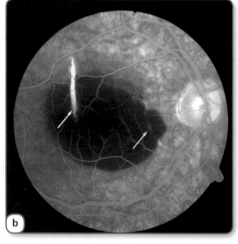

**Figure 69.3** Fluorescein angiography of choroidal rupture (corresponding to Figure 69.2). Two choroidal rupture sites with shallow overlying subretinal hemorrhage are shown (a) with corresponding fluorescein angiogram (b). There is significant blockage from the hemorrhage, and both choroidal rupture sites show bright staining (arrows), although the smaller rupture site (yellow arrow) is less apparent. Courtesy of Jeffrey Heier, MD.

with secondary stretching of the various, relatively elastic, portions of the eye (sclera, retina, vitreous). The relatively inelastic portions of the eye, such as the RPE layer, Bruch's membrane, and inner choroid are prone to rupture with blunt injuries. Choroidal rupture sites may be singular or multiple and most commonly occur in the posterior pole, particularly in the macula. Patient with pre-existing angioid streaks are more prone to the development of choroidal rupture due to the inherent weakness of Bruch's membrane in these patients.

## Symptoms and clinical findings

In cases with macular involvement or secondary subretinal hemorrhage involving the macula, decreased visual acuity is expected. There may be other associated ocular injuries, which can cause additional symptoms depending on the location, extent, and severity.

A choroidal rupture site has a characteristic appearance (Figure 69.1) with a crescenteric-shaped subretinal defect that is typically oriented in a roughly concentric orientation to the optic nerve, due to a relative binding effect of the RPE and Bruch's membrane concentrically to the edges of the nerve. Associated subretinal hemorrhage is common in the acute setting. Secondary choroidal neovascular membrane formation may occur later.

## Treatment/prognosis/follow-up

If submacular hemorrhage is obscuring a clear view of the tissue underlying the retina, waiting for the hemorrhage to improve spontaneously may be required to be able to make an accurate diagnosis. Pneumatic displacement of such a hemorrhage may also be considered, although it is not clear this management strategy offers a clear advantage, long-term, over conservative treatment. In the absence of a significant blunt traumatic event, where other external signs of periocular injury would be expected, other causes for submacular hemorrhage (such as choroidal neovascular membranes due to high myopia or age-related macular degeneration) should be considered.

Upon resolution of any secondary injuries or hemorrhage, visual acuity may return to normal if the fovea is spared or be permanently impaired to varying degrees if the macula is involved, which is more typical.

Secondary choroidal neovascular membrane formation following prior choroidal rupture occurs in approximately 5–10% of eyes and is more significant if the choroidal rupture involves the macula. Management of these membranes can be challenging, but they are usually most responsive to intravitreal anti-VEGF therapy.

## How to approach a patient with a preretinal hemorrhage overlying the macula

| Identify the primary pathologic clinical finding(s) | | |
|---|---|---|
| There is a large, layered, elevated preretinal hemorrhage that is obscuring the macula (**Figure 70.1**). | | |
| **Formulate a differential diagnosis** | | |
| **Most likely** | **Less likely** | **Least likely** |
| • Valsalva retinopathy | • Terson's syndrome, blood dyscrasia, leukemia | • Diabetic retinopathy, ruptured macroaneurysm, shaken baby syndrome |
| **Query patient history** | | |
| • Was there recent ocular trauma?<br>• Was there recent excessive straining against a closed glottis (i.e. coughing and vomiting)?<br>• Are there any systemic medical concerns? | | |
| **Decide on ancillary diagnostic imaging** | | |
| Optical coherence tomography (OCT) is useful to confirm the location of the hemorrhage, but in large hemorrhages there may be significant loss of signal posterior to the hemorrhage, limiting its application. Obtaining a vertical OCT scan on the edge of the hemorrhage provides the most useful information. Fluorescein angiography (FA) can be useful in the evaluation of various other entities being considered in the differential diagnosis. | | |

## Ancillary diagnostic imaging interpretation

### Optical coherence tomography

OCT shows hemorrhage located within the potential sub-internal limiting membrane (ILM) space (**Figure 70.2**). The hemorrhage appears as hyper-reflective material with significant shadowing artifact posteriorly. If visualized, the underlying retinal layers are intact and relatively undisturbed.

### Fluorescein angiography

FA would be expected to show blockage from the hemorrhage without any areas of hyperfluorescence.

### Color photography

Serial color photographs are useful to monitor for subtle changes in the hemorrhage over time, which can confirm spontaneous improvement.

## Final diagnosis: Valsalva retinopathy

### Epidemiology/etiology

Significant straining against a closed glottis provides the forces necessary to rupture capillaries on the surface of the retina, which allows Valsalva retinopathy to develop. Any physical activities where excessive straining occurs in the presence of a closed glottis can result in this condition. Such activities include coughing, vomiting, straining

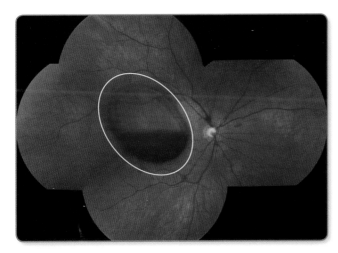

**Figure 70.1** Color photographs of Valsalva retinopathy. There is a layered preretinal hemorrhage (within yellow oval) obscuring the macula with a red-colored dependent portion rich in red blood cells inferiorly, and a relatively clear serous component superiorly.

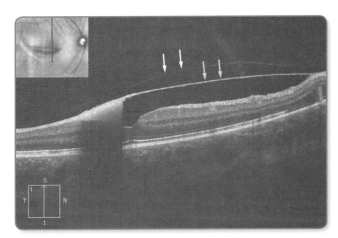

**Figure 70.2** Optical coherence tomography (OCT) of Valsalva retinopathy. A vertical line OCT shows residual hemorrhage (red arrows), which is located in the sub-ILM space. The posterior hyaloid (white arrows) and ILM (yellow arrows) are both clearly identifiable.

with bowel movements, lifting heavy objects, bungee jumping, playing contact sports, and child labor. The condition is typically unilateral but may be bilateral.

## Symptoms and clinical findings

Affected patients experience the sudden, painless loss of central vision, often associated with an identifiable event that included significant physical straining.

The hemorrhage will occupy and physically detach the sub-ILM potential space in a characteristic configuration (**Figure 70.1**). With time, the red blood cells layer dependently leaving a serous component superiorly. Breakthrough vitreous hemorrhage may develop.

## Treatment/prognosis/follow-up

The hemorrhage associated with Valsalva retinopathy invariable resorbs spontaneously if given enough time, typically within 6 months from onset. Upon resolution, no significant adverse effects to the underlying retina are expected and full visual recovery is typical. Nd:YAG laser membranotomy and surgical intervention with vitrectomy are two invasive options for treatment that can be considered in select cases, particularly when waiting a number of months for spontaneous visual improvement is not practical. Any potential medical conditions that may mimic Valsalva retinopathy should be excluded, particularly when an appropriate inciting event is not elicited in the patient's history.

## How to approach a patient with scattered bilateral white spots in the posterior pole

| Identify the primary pathologic clinical finding(s) | | |
|---|---|---|
| There are numerous patchy, fluffy, white, polygonally shaped lesions in the retina that resemble cotton-wool spots in a pattern located around the optic nerve and involving the macula bilaterally (**Figure 71.1**). | | |
| **Formulate a differential diagnosis** | | |
| **Most likely** | **Less likely** | **Least likely** |
| • Purtscher's retinopathy, Purtscher's-like retinopathy | • Diabetic retinopathy, hypertensive retinopathy | • Cytomegalovirus (CMV) retinitis, multiple evanescent white dot syndrome, acute posterior multifocal placoid pigment epitheliopathy |
| **Query patient history** | | |
| • Has there been significant recent trauma to the head, chest, or pelvis?<br>• Are there any significant systemic ailments such as pancreatitis or HIV?<br>• What is the patients' blood pressure? | | |
| **Decide on ancillary diagnostic imaging** | | |
| Although, the diagnosis is typically made on clinical grounds alone, fluorescein angiography (FA) can reveal characteristic patterns of blockage and/or leakage in various conditions being considered in the differential diagnosis. Optical coherence tomography (OCT) can also provide useful ancillary information to help confirm the diagnosis. | | |

## Ancillary diagnostic imaging interpretation

### Optical coherence tomography

OCT can provide information about the severity and location of macular involvement. Purtscher flecken, or characteristic patches of retinal whitening, have a characteristic appearance (**Figure 71.2**) that is pathognomonic of Purthscher's retinopathy.

### Fluorescein angiography

The appearance on FA varies with severity. There may be areas of hypofluorescence correlating with the patches of intraretinal whitening early and diffuse leakage from the retinal vasculature in the later phase (**Figure 71.3**). In more severe cases, there may be areas of complete arterial nonperfusion.

## Final diagnosis: Purtscher's retinopathy

### Epidemiology/etiology

Purtscher's or Purtscher's-like retinopathy is a rare occlusive vasculopathy that may occur following significant head, chest, or long-bone trauma or be seen in the setting of various medical conditions including acute pancreatitis and others. The findings are bilateral in the majority of cases. Traditionally, Purtscher's retinopathy has been

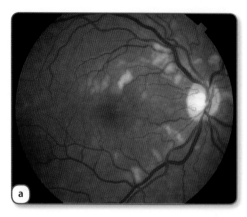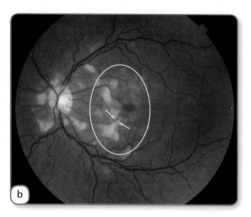

**Figure 71.1** Color photograph of Purtscher's retinopathy. Both eyes show typical features including numerous multilateral patches of intraretinal whitening or Purtscher flecken (within yellow circle). Within patches of retinal whitening, there are unaffected zones surrounding retinal arterioles (between arrows), which are pathognomonic of Purtscher's retinopathy.

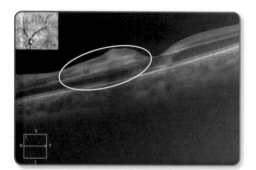

**Figure 71.2** Optical coherence tomography of Purtscher's retinopathy. Line scan through a Purtscher flecken reveals retinal hyper-reflectivity or edema of all of the inner retinal layers (circle), which are supplied by the retinal arterial circulation. This OCT appearance supports the mechanism of an occlusive retinal arterial process being implicated in Purtscher's retinopathy.

reserved for cases involving trauma, whereas when other etiologies cause a similar clinical picture the term Purtscher's-like retinopathy is more accurately used. The underlying mechanism for the clinical findings seen in both Purtscher's and Purtscher's-like retinopathy are thought to be similar although they are not clearly understood. Complement-mediated leukoembolization, fat embolism, or even angiospasm causing multiple arterial occlusions have been proposed as potential etiologic factors that cause the characteristic clinical findings, although no mechanism has been proven.

## Symptoms and clinical findings

The degree of and presence of vision loss can be variable. Intraretinal whitening resembling multiple, large cotton-wool spots in a pattern roughly circumscribing the optic nerve are typical. Some of these patches of retinal whitening are cotton-wool spots, while others are more accurately termed Purtscher flecken. There also may be intraretinal hemorrhages. Purtscher flecken are a pathognomonic description of retinal whitening with an uninvolved zone surrounding

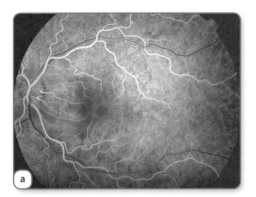

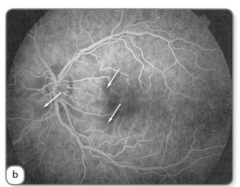

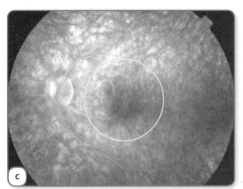

**Figure 71.3** Fluorescein angiography of Purtscher's retinopathy. Early (a) and mid (b) phase angiograms show patchy hypofluorescence due to blockage from the areas of retinal whitening (arrows). Later phase angiogram (c) shows leakage from retinal arterioles and venules (circle).

retinal arterioles or venules that are traversing through the affected retina (Figure 71.1). Their OCT appearance of inner retinal layer hyper-reflectivity supports the suggested pathophysiological mechanism of retinal capillary occlusion (Figure 71.2) and is in contrast to isolated hyper-reflectivity within the nerve fiber layer, which is the OCT appearance typical of cotton-wool spots.

## Treatment/prognosis/follow-up

There is no treatment with proven efficacy in any large controlled trials. There are isolated case reports of systemic corticosteroids being used with successful outcomes but this does not necessarily reflect any additional benefit over the natural history of the disease. Spontaneous improvement of vision is common along with resolution of the clinical features of disease over weeks to months after the initial injury or illness. Observation is the most typical course of action in this condition.

# Further reading

Agrawal A, McKibbin M. Purtscher's retinopathy: epidemiology, clinical features and outcome. Br J Ophthalmol 2007; 91:1456–9.

Miguel AI, Henriques F, Azevedo LF, Loureiro AJ, Maberley DA. Systematic review of Purtscher's and Purtscher-like retinopathies. Eye (Lond) 2013; 27:1–13.

## How to approach a patient with an unusual appearing crystalline lens

| Identify the primary pathologic clinical finding(s) | | |
|---|---|---|
| There is a dark, irregular shaped discoloration that appears embedded within the crystalline lens (**Figure 72.1**). | | |
| **Formulate a differential diagnosis** | | |
| **Most likely** | **Less likely** | **Least likely** |
| • Intralenticular foreign body | • Traumatic cataract | • Age-related cataract |
| **Query patient history** | | |
| • Has there been any recent trauma?<br>• Has the patient been working with metal recently (i.e. metal on metal hammering)?<br>• Has there been any recent pain involving the affected eye?<br>• Is the other eye affected by a similar problem? | | |
| **Decide on ancillary diagnostic imaging** | | |
| In the setting of a suspected intraocular foreign body, but where one is not clinically visible, ultrasonography and/or high-resolution computed tomography with thin slices are helpful in identifying an occult foreign body. If an occult metallic intraocular foreign body is suspected and signs of siderosis are present, electrophysiologic testing may be useful. | | |

## Ancillary diagnostic imaging interpretation

None.

## Final diagnosis: intralenticular foreign body

### Epidemiology/etiology

Intraocular foreign bodies occur in the setting of trauma and may be composed of organic or nonorganic material. The most frequently encountered type of intraocular foreign body is a small metallic fragment that fractured during grinding or hammering metal on metal. Intraocular foreign bodies occur in a minority of open globe injuries, more commonly in the setting of high-speed projectile injuries. The foreign body may be embedded in the cornea, lens, or retina or be located in the anterior chamber or vitreous cavity. About a quarter of intraocular foreign bodies are located in the anterior segment or lens (**Figure 72.1a**) with the remainder being present in the posterior segment (**Figure 72.2**).

### Symptoms and clinical findings

In the setting of a self-sealed entry wound, a patient may report no current ocular complaints but a recent history of ocular discomfort that has since resolved. Alternatively, if there are significant concurrent ocular injuries, there may be a severe impairment of vision, pain, photophobia, and other symptoms.

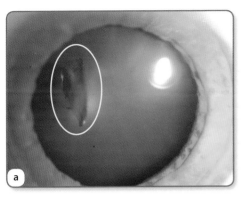 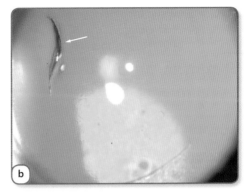

**Figure 72.1** Intralenticular foreign body. (a) Slit lamp photograph of a metallic fragment embedded within the crystalline lens (within yellow circle). (b) Slit lamp photograph with retroillumination highlights a self-sealed corneal laceration (arrow). This photograph was taken after combined cataract extraction, foreign body removal and intraocular lens placement from an anterior approach.

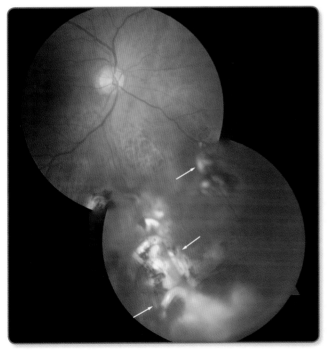

**Figure 72.2** Retained intraocular foreign body. This patient reported a remote history of an injury when a metal object exploded near his face. There is a corkscrew-shaped object embedded within the retina (arrows) that may be a metallic spring. No signs of siderosis were present and the patient was observed.

Clinical findings may include the direct identification of an intraocular foreign body, particularly if present in the anterior segment. Posteriorly located foreign bodies may also be directly visualized but are more frequently obscured by overlying media opacity, such as vitreous hemorrhage, due to concurrent injuries to nearby ocular structures. An associated entry wound is also typically identified. If an occult intraocular metallic foreign body has been present and missed for a period of time, features of siderosis may be present such as nyctalopia, iris heterochromia, peripheral retinal degeneration, cataract, or a poorly reactive pupil.

## Treatment/prognosis/follow-up

A thorough ophthalmic examination including slit lamp biomicroscopy, gonioscopy, and indirect ophthalmoscopy should be performed to identify any potential occult intraocular foreign body or other associated traumatic ocular injury. Particular attention should be focused on identification of any conjunctival/scleral laceration, corneal laceration, traumatic cataract, or iris irregularities. Very small wounds in the cornea can self-seal making them challenging to identify (**Figure 72.1b**).

When identified in the acute setting, intraocular foreign bodies of any type should be removed surgically to reduce the risk of endophthalmitis and other potential adverse toxic effects. Timing for removal of intraocular foreign bodies is somewhat controversial but, in general, prompt removal is indicated. Open globes should be repaired expeditiously to reduce the incidence of endophthalmitis, but foreign body removal can potentially be delayed until after primary globe closure, particularly if appropriately trained staff are unavailable. Retained intraocular foreign bodies identified at a time significantly removed from the initial trauma can be observed if the foreign body is composed of an inert material. If the material is unknown, careful observation for any early signs of a significant foreign body reaction such as siderosis is prudent and serial electroretinograms can be helpful.

## Further reading

Parke DW 3rd, Flynn HW Jr, Fisher YL. Management of intraocular foreign bodies: a clinical flight plan. Can J Ophthalmol 2013; 48:8–12.

# Nonaccidental trauma (shaken baby syndrome)

## How to approach a pediatric patient with multiple scattered retinal hemorrhages in the retina

| Identify the primary pathologic clinical finding(s) | | |
| --- | --- | --- |
| There are numerous retinal hemorrhages distributed diffusely throughout the fundus of both eyes (**Figure 73.1**). | | |
| **Formulate a differential diagnosis** | | |
| Most likely | Less likely | Least likely |
| • Shaken baby syndrome | • Birth-related trauma, Terson's syndrome, Valsalva retinopathy, leukemia, other blood dyscrasia | • Bilateral central retinal vein occlusions, Purtscher's syndrome, retinopathy of prematurity |
| **Query patient history** | | |
| • Are there any other systemic injuries that are consistent with child abuse (skull, rib, or long-bone fractures in various stages of healing, unexplained bruising, etc.)?<br>• Was there any recent accidental traumatic injury?<br>• Is the child in the presence of any other caregivers besides the parents?<br>• Are there any other symptoms or signs of systemic disease such as failure to thrive, poor feeding, weight loss, rashes, or pale skin? | | |
| **Decide on ancillary diagnostic imaging** | | |
| Color photographs are important to document findings. Fluorescein angiography (FA) can be useful if the diagnosis is in question but is difficult to obtain in young children and infants without general anesthesia and is generally not necessary. | | |

## Ancillary diagnostic imaging interpretation

### Fluorescein angiography

FA shows areas of hypofluorescence due to blockage from retinal hemorrhages that are present.

### Color photography

Color photographs are essential for documentation purposes, as these cases often will have significant medical–legal ramifications.

## Final diagnosis: shaken baby syndrome (nonaccidental trauma)

### Epidemiology/etiology

Shaken baby syndrome is a type of inflicted traumatic brain injury with a constellation of clinical injuries involving multiple organ systems, of which the ocular findings are very characteristic and important, when present, in contributing to the correct diagnosis. This is a rare condition associated with purposeful violent shaking or other inflicted head injury

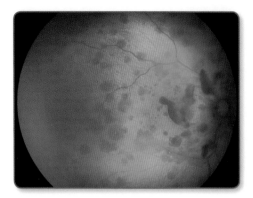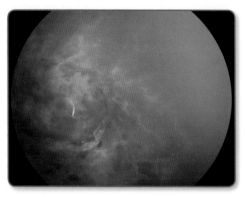

**Figure 73.1** Color RetCam photographs of shaken baby syndrome. There are many scattered hemorrhages in all retinal layers (pre-, intra-, and subretinal) throughout the fundi in both eyes, to a lesser degree in the right eye (a) compared to the left eye (b). Many of the retinal hemorrhages have a white center, which is typical. These images were from a 2-month-old infant, a victim of child abuse, who succumbed to his systemic injuries.

to an infant or young child and caries a significant risk of mortality. The pathogenesis for the retinal hemorrhages is not clear but thought to be related to acceleration/deceleration shearing forces between the vitreous and the retina or due to increases in retinal venous pressure. The history offered by the patients' family member or caretaker is often mismatched with the identified injuries.

## Symptoms and clinical findings

Affected patients are usually too young to verbalize any visual problems. Other concurrent systemic injuries coexistent with shaken baby syndrome may cause symptoms such as malaise or poor feeding and signs such as skin bruising or fractured bones may be present.

Clinical ophthalmic findings can vary in severity but are usually isolated to the retina and vitreous and have a distinguishing pattern from other etiologies. Many scattered pre-, intra-, and subretinal hemorrhages throughout the entire fundus of various shapes and sizes are typical, which may be characteristically dome shaped. Other clinical findings may include macular folds, retinoschisis, and breakthrough vitreous hemorrhage. The majority of cases are bilateral but may be asymmetric and, in rare cases, even unilateral. There usually are not any signs of direct external ocular or periocular trauma such as periorbital ecchymosis or subconjunctival hemorrhage. Other systemic injuries that may be concurrent with the ocular findings include intracranial hemorrhages (typically subdural), bruising, and fractures of the skull, ribs, or long bones (often in various stages of healing). The distinct clinical pattern of retinal hemorrhages along with the other systemic clinical findings help to distinguish shaken baby syndrome from any of the other considerations listed in the differential diagnosis.

## Treatment/prognosis/follow-up

A high index of suspicion for shaken baby syndrome should be maintained in any cases of unexplained retinal hemorrhages in an infant or young child. Patients are typically managed in an inpatient setting with a multidisciplinary team. Appropriate and expeditious notification to child protective services should be made if child abuse is suspected. Correct diagnosis is critical, particularly in milder cases where further abuse can be prevented, given the high mortality rate (about 30%) and associated morbidity with shaken baby syndrome. The severity of retinal hemorrhages generally correlates with the degree of concurrent brain injury and general prognosis.

# Further reading

Mungan NK. Update on shaken baby syndrome: ophthalmology. Curr Opin Ophthalmol 2007; 18:392–7.

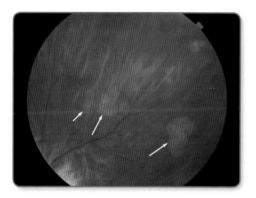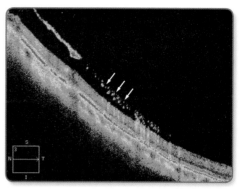

**Figure 74.2** Emulsified silicone oil on the retinal surface. (a) Multiple patches of fine emulsified silicone droplets are visible on the surface of the retina (arrows), trapped between the silicone oil interface and thin aqueous layer along the surface of the retina. (b) Optical coherence tomography of emulsified silicone oil droplets on the edge of the silicone oil interface (arrows).

reduction include maximizing the silicone oil fill and the inclusion of an encircling scleral buckle, although there is no clinical evidence that these strategies actually demonstrate any advantage. There is also experimental evidence that less viscous silicone oil (i.e. 1000 centistoke vs. 5000 centistoke) is more prone to emulsification, but this has also not been demonstrated clinically.

# Further reading

de Silva DJ, Lim KS, Schulenburg WE. An experimental study on the effect of encircling band procedure on silicone oil emulsification. Br J Ophthalmol 2005; 89:1348–50.
Heidenkummer HP, Kampik A, Thierfelder S. Emulsification of silicone oils with specific physicochemical characteristics. Graefes Arch Clin Exp Ophthalmol 1991; 229:88–94.
Scott IU, Flynn HW Jr, Murray TG, et al. Outcomes of complex retinal detachment repair using 1000- vs. 5000-centistoke silicone oil. Arch Ophthalmol 2005; 123:473–8.

## How to approach a patient with multiple clear liquid bubbles in the anterior chamber

| Identify the primary pathologic clinical finding(s) | | |
|---|---|---|
| There are many spherical, clear, liquid bubbles layered in the inferior portion of the anterior chamber (**Figure 75.1**). | | |
| **Formulate a differential diagnosis** | | |
| **Most likely** | **Less likely** | **Least likely** |
| • Retained perfluorocarbon liquid (PFCL) | • Emulsified silicone oil, cholesterolosis | • Uveitis |
| **Query patient history** | | |
| • Has the patient had prior vitreoretinal surgery? If so, was a complex retinal detachment present that required use of heavy liquids?<br>• Has the patient had prior ocular trauma? | | |
| **Decide on ancillary diagnostic imaging** | | |
| This is a diagnosis that is typically made on clinical grounds only. If retained perfluorocarbon is present subretinally, optical coherence tomography (OCT) can be helpful to confirm the diagnosis. | | |

## Ancillary diagnostic imaging interpretation

### Optical coherence tomography

OCT of subretinal perfluorocarbon reveals a round-shaped, hyporeflective, subretinal cavity with the overlying retina molding and conforming to its shape.

## Final diagnosis: retained PFCL

### Epidemiology/etiology

PFCL is a clear, dense liquid used intraoperatively during complex retinal detachment repair as a tool to assist in retinal flattening. After use, the liquid is removed, but not infrequently varying amounts may be unintentionally left in the eye. In rare cases, PFCL has been intentionally left in the eye in large amounts for retinal tamponade. Since such amounts invariably cause inflammation, planned removal is indicated no later than 2–3 weeks. Retained PFCL can be located in the anterior chamber (**Figure 75.1**), subretinally (**Figure 75.2**), or in the posterior chamber (**Figure 75.3**). The presence of retained PFCL is usually only recognized during postoperative examination.

### Symptoms and clinical findings

Depending on the location of the retained PFCL, various symptoms may be present. Perfluorocarbon in the anterior chamber or posterior chamber may lead to various optical aberrations and reflections that can be visualized by the patient. Subretinal perfluorocarbon may cause

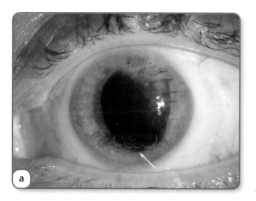
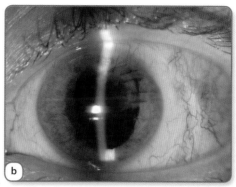

**Figure 75.1** Perfluorocarbon liquid in the anterior chamber. (a) There is retained perfluorocarbon liquid in the anterior chamber (yellow arrow) following repair of a complex traumatic retinal detachment. (b) Appearance of the same eye following removal of the perfluorocarbon liquid with a 25-gauge needle and syringe via an inferior limbal approach at the slit lamp biomicroscope. Courtesy of Jeffrey Heier, MD.

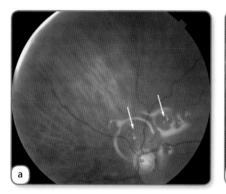
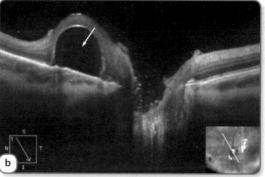

**Figure 75.2** Subretinal perfluorocarbon liquid. (a) A color photograph of retained subretinal perfluorocarbon located outside the macula (arrows). (b) Corresponding optical coherence tomography confirms the subretinal location and reveals a characteristic sharply circumscribed, roughly spherical, hyporeflective cavity, which corresponds to the perfluorocarbon liquid bubble (arrow). Courtesy of Caroline Baumal, MD.

a central or paracentral scotoma if located in the macula. Retained perfluorocarbon has a characteristic appearance, depending on location (**Figures 75.1–75.3**). Associated intraocular inflammation or elevated intraocular pressure may be present.

## Treatment/prognosis/follow-up

Identification of residual perfluorocarbon intraoperatively and removal during the initial surgery is the optimal course of action. If there is a small amount of retained PFCL present postoperatively in the absence of any secondary complications, indefinite observation is often appropriate. When significant amounts of PFCL are present in the anterior or posterior chamber, surgical removal is usually indicated to relieve symptoms and reduce risk of potential toxicity. This is usually

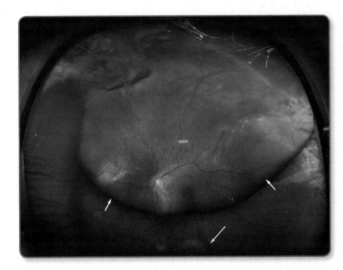

**Figure 75.3** Perfluorocarbon liquid in the posterior chamber (corresponds to Figure 75.1). Following complex retinal detachment repair in the setting of traumatic hemorrhagic choroidal detachments, silicone oil was used as a tamponade agent. An underfill of the silicone oil is evident (white arrows), which is a result of resolution of the choroidal detachments over time. Retained perfluorocarbon liquid is located inferiorly (yellow arrow), due to its higher density and specific gravity compared to both silicone oil and aqueous humor. Courtesy of Jeffrey Heier, MD.

performed by vitrectomy with active extrusion of the liquid. In cases of subretinal perfluorocarbon involving the macula, removal may be considered if there is a significant impairment to visual acuity, usually only if the fovea is involved. Various techniques for removal exist including subretinal bleb formation with direct removal or displacement of the heavy liquid outside of the macula. Techniques to minimize the occurrence of subretinal perfluorocarbon include a controlled, steady injection speed to minimize small bubble formation (which increases the risk of subretinal migration) and injecting within the bubble of perfluorocarbon that is already in the eye to maintain one large bubble. Small amounts of anterior chamber PFCL can be aspirated at the slit lamp with a needle via a paracentesis.

# Further reading

Suk KK, Flynn HW Jr. Management options for submacular perfluorocarbon liquid. Ophthalmic Surg Lasers Imaging 2011; 42:284–91.
Roth DB, Sears JE, Lewis H. Removal of retained subfoveal perfluoro-n-octane liquid. Am J Ophthalmol 2004; 138:287–9.

# 76

# Globe perforation from local anesthesia

## How to approach a patient with subretinal and vitreous hemorrhage immediately following cataract surgery

| Identify the primary pathologic clinical finding(s) | | |
| --- | --- | --- |
| There is vitreous hemorrhage overlying subretinal hemorrhage and the globe is hypotonus (**Figure 76.1**). | | |
| **Formulate a differential diagnosis** | | |
| **Most likely** | **Less likely** | **Least likely** |
| • Globe perforation from periorbital anesthetic administration | • Suprachoroidal hemorrhage | • Rhegmatogenous retinal detachment |
| **Query patient history** | | |
| • Is the patient highly myopic with a posterior staphyloma? <br> • What kind of anesthesia was provided during their recent ocular surgery? <br> • Did the patient experience sudden pain or loss of vision during periorbital anesthesia administration for their recent ocular surgery? <br> • Were any abnormalities identified during their surgery such as loss of the red reflex? | | |
| **Decide on ancillary diagnostic imaging** | | |
| If the vitreous hemorrhage is severe, ultrasonography is indicated to evaluate the underlying retina. If there is macular involvement, optical coherence tomography (OCT) can provide useful information. | | |

## Ancillary diagnostic imaging interpretation

### Optical coherence tomography

Particularly in the setting of a double perforation, the macula may be affected. In such a case, OCT can provide insight into the severity of the macular injury and help provide prognostic information (**Figure 76.2**).

## Final diagnosis: globe perforation from periorbital anesthesia

### Epidemiology/etiology

Globe penetration or perforation may occur unintentionally during peribulbar or retrobulbar anesthesia during ocular surgery at a roughly equivalent rate. This complication is exceedingly rare with an incidence of about 0.1% but can be potentially devastating. Risk factors associated with an increased incidence include eyes that are highly myopic with posterior staphyloma, delivery of multiple injections, and poor patient cooperation. At the time of occurrence, this complication often goes unrecognized and is often only suspected during examination on the first postoperative day. The most common location for globe perforation is the inferotemporal quadrant.

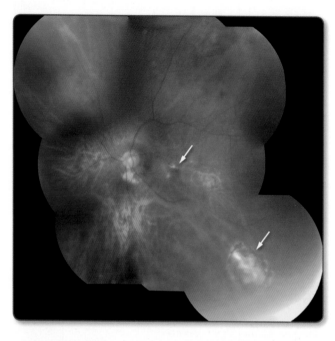

**Figure 76.1** Color photograph of double globe perforation secondary to retrobulbar anesthesia. This patient initially presented with vitreous hemorrhage and inferior subretinal hemorrhage 1 day following uncomplicated cataract extraction with intraocular lens placement, performed with a retrobulbar anesthetic block. Prompt vitrectomy was performed, and intraoperatively, double perforation sites were identified. The entry site is in the inferotemporal periphery and exit site is in the macula (arrows). The subretinal hemorrhage was evacuated and the retina was flatted. This photograph was taken 6 weeks postoperatively. Courtesy of Caroline Baumal, MD.

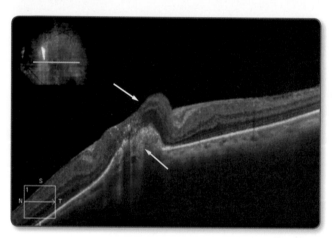

**Figure 76.2** Optical coherence tomography of globe perforation involving the macula (corresponding to Figure 76.1). There is significant submacular scarring (yellow arrow) and distortion of the overlying retinal layers (white arrow) in the vicinity of the fovea. Courtesy of Caroline Baumal, MD.

## Symptoms and clinical findings

Symptoms include sudden onset of pain and/or loss of vision. Clinical findings include loss of the red reflex during surgery, unexplained hypotony, vitreous hemorrhage, subretinal hemorrhage, retinal tear, retinal detachment, and in very rare cases even globe rupture. A single or double perforation site may be identified (Figure 76.1).

## Treatment/prognosis/follow-up

Strategies to minimize the occurrence of this complication are important to consider when administering periorbital anesthesia such as peribulbar or retrobulbar injections. These measures include using the minimum needle length necessary (1.25 inches for peribulbar and 1.5 inches for retrobulbar), having the patient maintain straight ahead gaze, and a comprehensive understanding of the involved anatomy. Using alternative anesthesia modalities such as topical anesthesia, sub-Tenon anesthesia, or general anesthesia eliminate the possibility of this complication.

Subspecialist vitreoretinal referral should be made promptly if globe perforation is suspected. Management strategies are tailored to the type and extent of injury. Some perforation sites may self-seal and be managed with observation only or localized retinopexy if indicated. In the setting of significant vitreous hemorrhage, retinal detachment, or globe rupture, prompt surgical intervention is indicated (**Figure 76.3**).

Prognosis is poor if retinal detachment is present on detection of a globe perforation resulting from periorbital anesthesia, with final visual acuity unlikely to extend beyond counting fingers. If a retinal detachment is not present initially, prognosis is better, although it can be variable.

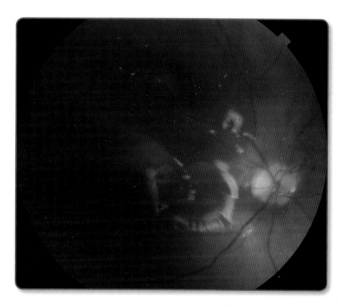

**Figure 76.3**  Color photograph following surgical repair of globe rupture secondary to peribulbar anesthetic block. This patient was scheduled to undergo vitrectomy with membrane peeling for an epiretinal membrane. During peribulbar block administration, there was immediate concern for globe perforation due to eye pain, loss of red reflex, and hypotony prompting referral to our institution. Surgical exploration revealed a large scleral laceration with globe rupture, which was repaired. Concurrent vitrectomy was performed, which revealed vitreous hemorrhage, complex retinal detachment, and subretinal hemorrhage. The retina was reattached and silicone oil was used for tamponade. This photograph shows the postoperative appearance of the macula with some persistent subretinal hemorrhage.

# Further reading

Duker JS, Belmont JB, Benson WE, et al. Inadvertent globe perforation during retrobulbar and peribulbar anesthesia. Patient characteristics, surgical management, and visual outcome. Ophthalmology 1991; 98:519–26.

Ginsburg RN, Duker JS. Globe perforation associated with retrobulbar and peribulbar anesthesia. Semin Ophthalmol 1993; 8:87–95.

Schrader WF, Schargus M, Schneider E, Josifova T. Risks and sequelae of scleral perforation during peribulbar or retrobulbar anesthesia. J Cataract Refract Surg 2010; 36:885–9.

# Suprachoroidal hemorrhage

## How to approach a patient with the sudden development of a dark, elevated area involving the peripheral retina

| Identify the primary pathologic clinical finding(s) | | |
|---|---|---|
| There is a darkly colored, dome-shaped elevation underneath the peripheral/equatorial retina (**Figure 77.1**). | | |
| **Formulate a differential diagnosis** | | |
| **Most likely** | **Less likely** | **Least likely** |
| • Spontaneous suprachoroidal hemorrhage | • Choroidal melanoma | • Choroidal nevus, retinal detachment, posterior scleritis |
| **Query patient history** | | |
| • Has there been recent intraocular surgery?<br>• Has there been recent ocular trauma?<br>• Is the patient experiencing any eye pain?<br>• How old is the patient? | | |
| **Decide on ancillary diagnostic imaging** | | |
| If a small suprachoroidal hemorrhage is present, a number of imaging modalities can be used to help confirm the diagnosis including optical coherence tomography (OCT), fluorescein and indocyanine green angiography (ICGA), fundus autofluorescence (FAF), and ultrasonography. In more severe cases, particularly where there is significant anterior segment media opacity, ancillary testing is typically limited to ultrasonography. | | |

## Ancillary diagnostic imaging interpretation

### Optical coherence tomography

OCT is particularly useful if a scan can be performed on the edge of the area of interest, incorporating a normal area of the retina and the involved region. A suprachoroidal hemorrhage can be localized to the space between the choroid and sclera on OCT (**Figure 77.2**), which helps to differentiate this from other entities such as a choroidal melanoma or retinal detachment.

### Fluorescein angiography and indocyanine green angiography

Fluorescein angiography and ICGA show either a fairly normal retinal and choroidal circulation or general hypofluorescence in the area of the lesion (**Figure 77.3**). No double circulation or speckled hyperfluorescence is present, as might be seen in choroidal melanoma.

### Fundus autofluorescence

There is blocked or hypoautofluorescence on FAF imaging in the location of a suprachoroidal hemorrhage (**Figure 77.4**).

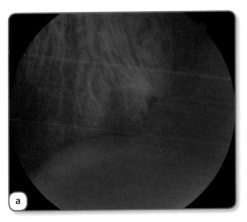 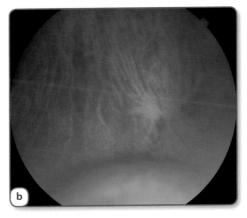

**Figure 77.1** Small, spontaneous suprachoroidal hemorrhage. There is a characteristic darkly colored, dome-shaped elevation underneath the peripheral retina. Differentiation of this lesion from a choroidal melanoma is not certain based on clinical grounds alone.

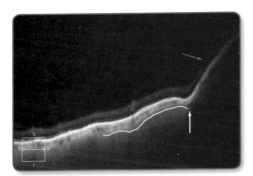

**Figure 77.2** Optical coherence tomography (corresponding to Figure 77.1). Normal retina, retinal pigment epithelium (RPE), choroid, and sclera are seen left of the white arrow with clear distinction of the choroid–sclera junction (yellow line). To the right of the arrow, there is loss of scleral details with a hyporeflective dome-shaped elevation due to suprachoroidal hemorrhage. The overlying retina, RPE, and choroid can still be seen (red arrow), but not the sclera, which has been mechanically pushed out of view by the hemorrhage.

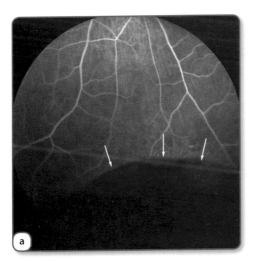 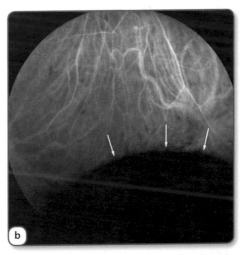

**Figure 77.3** Fluorescein (a) and indocyanine green (b) angiography. Both angiographic imaging modalities show hypofluorescence corresponding to the suprachoroidal hemorrhage (arrows), which is sharply demarcated from the uninvolved area.

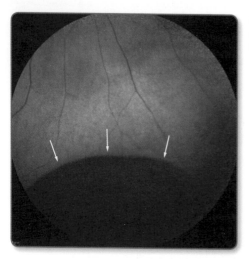

**Figure 77.4** Fundus autofluorescence. The area corresponding to the suprachoroidal hemorrhage (arrows) exhibits complete hypoautofluorescence.

## A- and B-scan ultrasonography

Ultrasonography is useful to confirm the diagnosis of suprachoroidal hemorrhage of any size. Once the diagnosis has been confirmed, ultrasound offers the most useful information in regards to severity and location of the hemorrhage and helps to monitor for any spontaneous improvement or worsening. B scan shows a highly reflective, irregular, potentially mobile, mass-like object within a choroidal detachment (**Figure 77.5**). Echographic patterns on A-scan ultrasound can help to

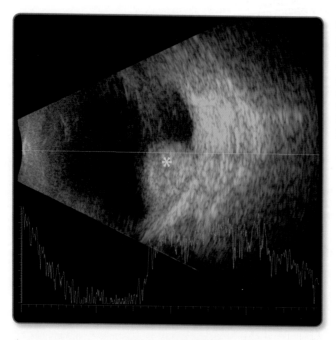

**Figure 77.5** Ultrasonography of a small, spontaneous suprachoroidal hemorrhage. This ultrasound demonstrates a characteristic dome-shaped elevation of the choroid (asterisk). The contents within the suprachoroidal space are highly reflective, consistent with hemorrhage.

differentiate serous from hemorrhagic choroidal detachments, if there is a question. Serous choroidals demonstrate minimal or no internal reflectivity and freshly hemorrhagic choroidals demonstrate high and irregular internal reflectivity. Both types of choroidal detachment demonstrate an initial wide and steep, double-peaked spike.

# Final diagnosis: suprachoroidal hemorrhage

## Epidemiology/etiology

Suprachoroidal hemorrhage is the development of blood in the potential suprachoroidal space, between the sclera and choroid. Suprachoroidal hemorrhages are rare, occurring in <1% of intraocular surgical procedures. They occur most commonly during or following recent intraocular surgery of any kind, although they may also occur after trauma or even spontaneously. In cases that occur due to surgery, the mechanism of suprachoroidal hemorrhage is presumed due to transient (or prolonged) hypotony with resultant rupture of blood vessels within the suprachoroidal space. The actual forces causing vascular rupture are likely a result of mechanical stretching due to changes in the globe wall that occur during hypotony. Risk factors for the development of a suprachoroidal hemorrhage include advanced age, hypertension, atherosclerosis, recent intraocular surgery, hypotony, and, possibly, concurrent use of anticoagulants.

## Symptoms and clinical findings

The size and extent of a suprachoroidal hemorrhage dictates both the symptoms and clinical findings. Symptoms may include decreased visual acuity, severe eye pain, nausea, and vomiting in severe cases.

Clinical findings depend on severity. Smaller suprachoroidal hemorrhages, more likely to occur spontaneously rather than following surgery, may be difficult to distinguish from other conditions such as choroidal melanoma and retinal detachment (**Figure 77.1**), with ancillary diagnostic testing being helpful to make the distinction. Larger suprachoroidal hemorrhages take on a characteristic four-lobed appearance due to choroid-sclera attachments at the vortex vein ampullae. Massive suprachoroidal hemorrhages are more common in the setting of intraocular surgery and can involve the entire circumference of the choroid. In extreme cases, the hemorrhage may be so bullous that there is apposition of inner retinal surfaces of opposite sides of the eye, termed 'kissing choroidals' (**Figure 77.6**).

## Treatment/prognosis/follow-up

A suprachoroidal hemorrhage is one of the most feared and, potentially, devastating surgical complications encountered by ophthalmologists. When occurring intraoperatively, they can result in expulsion of intraocular contents. Methods to reduce the incidence and severity of intraoperative suprachoroidal hemorrhages include minimization of hypotony and large intraocular pressure fluctuations, avoidance of

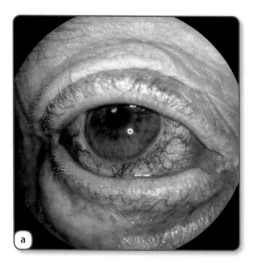 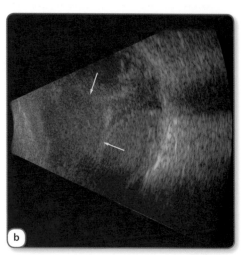

**Figure 77.6** Appositional suprachoroidal hemorrhage. (a) Anterior segment photograph shows flattening of the anterior chamber with iris-cornea touch. (b) Ultrasound demonstrates appositional or 'kissing' hemorrhagic choroidal detachments. Arrows identify locations of retinal apposition.

Valsalva maneuvers, and early recognition. Initial signs of a significant suprachoroidal hemorrhage during anterior segment surgery include loss of the red reflex, unexplained globe firmness, anterior prolapse of ocular contents, and rapid anterior chamber shallowing. Immediate closure of any open surgical wounds as soon as possible is critical to limit the extent of hemorrhage and prevent expulsion of intraocular contents. Subsequent surgical intervention to address suprachoroidal hemorrhage is controversial in regards to timing and indication. Generally, allowing 7–14 days for clot liquefaction is ideal to achieve optimal anatomical outcomes if surgical drainage is to be performed. Concomitant rhegmatogenous or tractional retinal detachment, retinal apposition, or severely elevated intraocular pressure may factor into a decision in favor of surgical intervention. The prognosis for large suprachoroidal hemorrhages is typically quite poor regardless of subsequent intervention. Smaller suprachoroidal hemorrhages, particularly those occurring spontaneously, tend to be more benign and can often be observed with spontaneous regression and a good prognosis.

# Further reading

Chu TG, Green RL. Suprachoroidal hemorrhage. Surv Ophthalmol 1999; 43:471–86.

# Index

Note: Page numbers in **bold** or *italic* refer to tables or figures, respectively.